Learning
Pharmacology
through
MCQ

D1514837

Benedict R. Lucchesi, Ph.D., M.D.
Department of Pharmacology
M 6322 Medical Science I
University of Michigan Medical School
Ann Arbor, Michigan 48109

Learning Pharmacology through MCQ

A Comprehensive Text

SECOND EDITION

B. J. Large and **I. E. Hughes**
Department of Pharmacology
University of Leeds, UK

JOHN WILEY & SONS
Chichester · New York · Brisbane · Toronto · Singapore

Other Wiley Editorial Offices

John Wiley & Sons, Inc., 605 Third Avenue,
New York, NY 10158-0012, USA

Jacaranda Wiley Ltd, G.P.O. Box 859, Brisbane,
Queensland 4001, Australia

John Wiley & Sons (Canada) Ltd, 22 Worcester Road,
Rexdale, Ontario M9W 1L1, Canada

John Wiley & Sons (SEA) Pte Ltd, 37 Jalan Pemimpin 05-04,
Block B, Union Industrial Building, Singapore 2057

Library of Congress Cataloging-in-Publication Data:

Large, B. J.
    Learning pharmacology through MCQ : a comprehensive text / B. J.
Large and I. E. Hughes.—2nd ed.
        p.   cm.
    ISBN 0 471 92708 2
        1. Pharmacology—Examinations, questions, etc.   I. Hughes, I. E.
II. Title.
    [DNLM: 1. Pharmacology—examination questions. QV 18 L322L]
    RM301.L37   1990
    615'.1'076—dc20
    DNLM/DLC   89-21548
    for Library of Congress   CIP

British Library Cataloguing in Publication Data

Large, B. J.
    Learning pharmacology through MCQ.—2nd ed.
    1. Pharmacology
    I. Title   II. Hughes, I. E.
    615.1

    ISBN 0 471 92708 2

Phototypeset by Dobbie Typesetting Limited, Plymouth, Devon
Printed and bound by Courier International Ltd, Tiptree, Essex

Contents

Contents

Preface

The multiple choice question (MCQ) in its variety of formats has become increasingly popular with examiners, especially of science undergraduates. There are many reasons for this surge of popularity: MCQs are objective in the assessment they provide, are consistent and are easily marked using, for example, computer marking techniques. Furthermore, the structure of scientific knowledge readily fits the MCQ formats.

We have found MCQs useful not just in examining students but also in *teaching*. They enable learning defects to be identified and deficiencies to be recognized; they give instant correction when answers are supplied and the teaching value is even greater if full explanations are provided along with the correct answers. From our considerable experience with such material in computer-aided tuition, we find students more appreciative and better informed when longer explanations are used which give the background to the topic being tested and set the question in context (as well as giving directly the answers to the specific questions).

The format of our MCQs is one that is frequently used in examinations and consists of a stem followed by five possible completions; each completed statement may be true (T) or false (F). One such question appears on each page and is followed by a commentary in which the correct answers may be discovered. The sequence of possible completions may not parallel the order in which the answers appear in any one commentary. At the end of the text will be found the correct answers in abbreviated form (e.g. TTFFF). On each page the names of individual drugs, but not groups or classes of drugs, are emphasized in bold type. There is a comprehensive index listing the names of all the chemicals mentioned and the question(s) in which they are referred to.

Students will approach this material in different ways. Some may attempt self-assessment of their knowledge in a particular area of pharmacology and to this end questions are grouped conventionally as in a systematic pharmacology course. Other students will assess their knowledge on questions chosen at random. However, many may decide to read one or a series of commentaries before attempting to answer the questions posed. To facilitate this approach each section begins with basic information, followed in later pages by additional material which builds on this knowledge. Thus consecutive commentaries may be used in the fashion of a textbook.

Learning Pharmacology through MCQ is intended for any medical or science student who needs to study pharmacology. Some questions focus attention on therapeutic and clinical areas while others relate to laboratory practice. We hope this book will also provide staff with ideas and material for use both in teaching and in examining.

The choice of material – its excesses, its deficiencies and its idiosyncracies – is entirely our responsibility, as is its accuracy. Some ambiguities may be found in certain questions but we feel this is less important when they are used for teaching purposes than if they were used for examinations. We hope the commentaries will at least show how we reached the answers that are provided.

Preface to the Second Edition

Our concept expressed in the first edition remains the same: namely, to provide students with an opportunity to learn or revise the subject of pharmacology and then to test their knowledge while acquiring skills in answering multiple choice questions.

Pharmacology is developing rapidly. New drugs are being introduced and older remedies supplanted. Hypotheses on how drugs act are being reformulated or fresh ones advanced. To bring the material up to date we have incorporated about 40 new pages and revised, sometimes substantially, most of the remainder. In the light of our experience and in response to comments from readers, the sections on peripheral and central nervous systems and endocrine pharmacology have been expanded; those on cardiovascular and blood now adjoin. Changes in the order of presentation have been made in most sections to improve continuity. We hope the next generation of readers will benefit accordingly.

We are grateful to friends, colleagues, reviewers and student readers who indicated ambiguities and errors in the first edition. We trust they are satisfied with our attempts to right them and hope they will notify us of the new ones created in the process of revision!

We acknowledge with thanks the help and unfailing courtesy of the editorial and production staff of John Wiley & Sons Ltd; the secretarial expertise of Miss Patricia Ritchie; and our wives for extending to us their patience during the 9-month gestation period of this book, as we did to them in previous similar periods.

Absorption, Distribution, Excretion and Biotransformation

MCQ 1

Drugs may be administered to man

1. orally and are then absorbed from the intestine and bypass the liver.
2. by inhalation only when a direct effect on the airways is required.
3. intravenously, though this is potentially hazardous since drug concentrations build up rapidly at the sites of action.
4. intramuscularly, when the high blood flow will permit rapid absorption of many drugs from aqueous solution.
5. intraperitoneally, a route commonly used in giving sedatives to violent schizophrenic patients.

An effective concentration of a drug must be achieved at its site of action in order that pharmacological effects can be produced. The chemical nature of the drug molecule will influence the speed at which this is achieved by affecting the drug's absorption, distribution, biotransformation and excretion.

Absorption of a drug into the body varies according to the route of administration and the ease with which the drug crosses cell membranes. Sometimes it may be desirable for a drug *not* to be absorbed into the bloodstream (e.g. treatment of intraluminal infections of the gut) but more usually drugs will be carried by the blood to their site of action. The oral route (p.o.) is most commonly used in clinical medicine, but in laboratory studies in other species routes are often chosen which are rarely used in man, such as intraperitoneal, used in man only to inject antiserum in the treatment of rabies. Administration p.o. is the most convenient and, for the majority of drugs, absorption is efficient because of the large surface area (around 4500 m^2) of the small intestine. However, drugs may be subjected to the acid and alkaline environments of the stomach and small intestine respectively, to the actions of intraluminal enzymes and, after passage to the liver in the portal blood, to the actions of the hepatic enzymes.

Some drugs taken into the mouth are absorbed from the buccal cavity (e.g. **glyceryl trinitrate**), thus circumventing the problems outlined above. Others are inhaled through the nose or mouth either for rapid absorption from the large alveolar surface of the lungs (e.g. gaseous anaesthetics: **amyl nitrite**) or to produce a local effect on the airways (e.g. sympathomimetic broncho-dilators: **sodium cromoglycate**). When formulated appropriately, some drugs may be administered transdermally. For instance, the glucocorticoid **flurandrenolide** may be applied through an impregnated sticky tape, permitting absorption through the skin. **Glyceryl trinitrate** may be applied once daily as a skin patch to prolong its antianginal activity and **scopolamine** is available in similar form to give an antiemetic effect for up to 3 days.

Alternative routes all require drugs to be injected and therefore the risks increase because vascular damage or infection may arise. Intravenous administration enables a high concentration of drug to be rapidly delivered. Intramuscular delivery can provide rapid absorption of water-soluble drugs or slow absorption from depot preparations in oil. Subcutaneous injections are given when great speed of absorption is not essential; generally only small volumes can be given. FFTTF

Diffusion into cells

1. of large water-soluble drug molecules requires their dissolution in membrane lipids.
2. occurs more readily with the ionized than the non-ionized form of weak electrolytes.
3. is more rapid with small water-soluble cations if they move from a positively to a negatively charged medium.
4. of weak electrolytes takes place with equal ease regardless of the pH of the medium.
5. is generally slow with lipid-soluble molecules that are too large to pass through the pores in cell membranes.

The majority of drugs must pass through several membranes to reach their site of action. An anxiolytic drug like **chlordiazepoxide** (given p.o.) must cross the gut and capillary walls, the 'blood–brain barrier' and possibly the cell walls of some CNS neurones. Further barriers would have to be crossed before the drug could be eliminated from the body. The mechanisms by which drugs cross membranes are diffusion (simple and facilitated), active transport and pinocytosis.

Cell membranes are made up of a bimolecular lipid layer with proteins and lipoproteins embedded in it. The fluidity of this layer enables pores to open, through which water-soluble substances may pass. There is a turnover of the membrane constituents (further contributing to its fluidity) which can result, for example, in changes in receptor density on the cell surface.

Drugs which are lipid-soluble can easily dissolve in the bilayer and move down their concentration gradient into the cell (and out again). However, a drug that is appreciably soluble only in water will move through the pores and the rate of passage will then be determined largely by molecular size. It must be noted that ions are water-soluble but, because they possess electrical charge, they can additionally be 'driven' across membranes (or prevented from moving) by the size of their charge and the potential difference between the two sides.

Most drugs are weak electrolytes and are partially dissociated in solution. The ionic form is less soluble in lipid (therefore crossing membranes with difficulty) than the non-ionized form. The pH of the solution will greatly affect the dissociation of weak electrolytes and hence their speed of absorption. A weak acid will ionize according to the equation

$$HA \rightleftharpoons H^+ + A^-$$

In an already acid medium the concentration of H^+ will be high and the equilibrium will therefore be pushed to the left. Thus the passage of a weak acid across a membrane will be enhanced the lower the pH of the solution since more will be in the uncharged form. The situation with a weak base is the reverse since less ionization occurs at a high pH so that transfer across membranes will be favoured from alkaline solutions.

Dissociation of weak acids and bases is characterized by a pK_a value (on a log scale, like pH) which is identical to the pH at which the weak electrolyte is 50% dissociated. A knowledge of pK_a values along with the chemical nature of drugs is useful because it enables the effect of pH changes on ionization to be predicted. TFTFF

3

MCQ 3

In considering the movement of weak electrolytes into cells

1. only the uncharged form is present inside the cell, as only this form penetrates the lipid membrane.
2. the dissociation of a weak acid increases as the pH falls, thereby increasing the rate of diffusion.
3. the equation $pH = pK_a + \log[A^-]/[HA]$ relates the degree of dissociation of a weak acid to the pH of the medium.
4. **strychnine** (a weak base) would be better absorbed from the stomach at lower pH values.
5. the renal excretion of a weak acid would be accelerated by acidification of the urine.

Diffusion involves movement of molecules down a concentration gradient. Water-soluble drugs generally cross membranes slowly because they must diffuse through pores which occupy only a fraction of the total area of membrane. Lipid-soluble drugs pass most readily because of their ability to dissolve in the lipid component forming the bulk of the cell membrane. The pH of a solution influences the ionization of a weak electrolyte and hence its passage across membranes since it is the non-ionized form of the molecule which is more lipid-soluble. Both forms are present inside the cell since the charged and non-charged forms exist in equilibrium. Some of the non-charged molecules which penetrate the cell membrane will ionize once inside to maintain the equilibrium.

The equations

$$pH = pK_a + \log[A^-]/[HA] \quad \text{and} \quad pH = pK_a + \log[B]/[BH^+]$$

illustrate the relationship for acids and bases respectively. It can be seen that the pK_a value is equal to the pH at which 50% ionization occurs because, when $[A^-] = [HA]$, then $pH = pK_a$ (since the log of 1 is zero).

When a weak acid, pK_a 6, is in solution at pH 7, then $\log[A^-]/[HA] = pH - pK_a = 1$. This means that the ratio $[A^-]/[HA]$ is 10; at pH 7 this acid will be 91% ionized, at pH 8 about 99% ionized and at pH 5 about 9% ionized. Thus even small changes of pH at values near to the pK_a of a drug will have a profound effect on the degree of ionization and therefore on lipid solubility. Similar calculations made for a weak base, pK_a 8, would show 99.9% ionization at pH 5 and 9% at pH 9.

The apparent harmlessness of the poison **strychnine** (weak base, pK_a about 8) when introduced in acid solution (pH 3) into the pylorically ligated stomach of the anaesthetized cat is due to its failure to be absorbed. Cats receiving the same dose in an alkaline medium died because of the increased proportion of lipid-soluble uncharged form, which accelerated the absorption into the bloodstream.

The above relationships are important in the treatment of various types of poisoning. The renal excretion of a weak base will be accelerated if the urine is made acid. Much of the drug will be filtered in the glomerulus and the filtrate will be concentrated in the tubules. The more acid the fluid in the lumen, the greater dissociation of the base and the smaller the concentration of the uncharged form which can diffuse back into the body through the tubule walls. In analogous fashion, the excretion of weak acids will be increased by alkalinization of the urine. FFTFF

The process of active transport moves substances across cell membranes and

1. requires energy which is generated by mitochondria within the cell.
2. is used only to propel molecules which are too large to penetrate by diffusion.
3. is able to move molecules against their concentration gradient.
4. can be blocked by drugs like **cyanide**.
5. often involves an (Na⁺, K⁺)-ATPase within the membrane, which can be inhibited by cardiac glycosides.

Usually drugs diffuse across cell membranes down their concentration gradients. Sometimes movement occurs faster than predicted without any additional energy expenditure by the membrane; this is called facilitated diffusion. It is thought to occur on carrier molecules which oscillate to and fro in the membrane and operates principally in the transfer of sugars, amino acids and drugs of similar chemical constitution. Its importance in drug absorption is not great. Tetracyclines are generally absorbed well from the gut but the possession of a specialized transporting mechanism by bacterial cells enables these drugs to exert a selectively toxic effect.

More common is another carrier-mediated system called active transport. This mechanism can move chemical substances *against* a concentration gradient (i.e. in the opposite direction from diffusion) and can also transport poorly diffusible substances down their concentration gradient. The process depends on metabolic energy generated by the membrane. If the supply of energy is blocked (e.g. by **cyanide**), then active transport ceases and a simple diffusion of material begins. Active transport is responsible for the maintenance of uneven concentrations of ions inside and outside cells. Sodium concentrations are higher outside than inside cells, while the reverse is true for potassium. Since these ions are constantly diffusing across membranes *down* their concentration gradients, the active transport system (or membrane pump) pumps sodium out and potassium back into the cell. In many cells it appears that the same mechanism is used for both movements so that as the carrier releases sodium to the outside of the cell it picks up a potassium ion and shuttles it inside.

The energy required is derived from the breakdown of ATP, in particular by the membrane enzyme called (Na⁺, K⁺)-ATPase, which requires the transported ions for activation. While this pump plays little part in the transfer of drugs, it is pharmacologically important because inhibition of the enzyme by drugs will affect ionic distribution and hence cellular function.

Cardiac glycosides such as **ouabain** inhibit (Na⁺, K⁺)-ATPase, particularly in cardiac tissue where these glycosides affect automaticity and excitability. These actions are thought to be dependent on enzyme inhibition, which secondarily affects the sequestration of intracellular calcium. FFTTT

MCQ 5

Absorption of drugs from the gut lumen

1. follows Fick's law.
2. occurs most readily from the small intestine because of its large surface area.
3. will not take place in the stomach if the drug is a weak electrolyte.
4. occurs at a faster rate in the presence of antispasmodic substances like **atropine**.
5. is increased if intestinal blood flow is increased.

The absorption of a drug from the gut lumen into the bloodstream is influenced by many factors including the chemical properties of the drug itself as well as the biological processes to which it is subjected.

A few substances like sugars, amino acids, **iron** and tetracyclines are absorbed by facilitated diffusion or active transport but the majority of absorbed drugs pass by simple diffusion. This can be depicted mathematically by a modification of Fick's formula:

$$T = kA\Delta C$$

where T is the amount of drug absorbed in unit time, k is a permeability constant of the membrane, A is the surface area involved and ΔC is the concentration gradient (the difference between the concentrations in the lumen and in capillary blood). Since the absorptive area of the small intestine is far greater than that of the stomach, the greatest proportion of most drugs is absorbed from the duodenum, jejunum and ileum. It must be borne in mind, however, that the strong acid in the stomach will suppress the ionization of weak acids, leaving the lipid-soluble uncharged form free to be absorbed from this region. The more complete ionization of weak bases in this acid environment may inhibit completely their absorption from the stomach. The change to the more alkaline environment of the duodenum will promote absorption of weakly basic drugs. Although ionization of weak acids will now be enhanced, the large surface area for absorption will enable a large proportion of such drugs to be absorbed from there in spite of the increased amount of the less lipid-soluble form. The human small intestine is about 6 m long, yet so folded is the luminal membrane (because of the villi and the brush border of epithelial cells) that its absorptive area is between 4000 and 5000 m^2.

About 25% of cardiac output goes to the gut and liver so the high blood flow rapidly transports away the molecules of absorbed drug, helping to maintain a high concentration gradient. Because many drugs bind to the plasma proteins (and are then no longer freely diffusible because of the molecular size of the complex), this further enhances the concentration gradient since only free drug contributes. In general, gut motility enhances absorption because it maintains a high blood flow, helps dissolution and mixing, and speeds gastric emptying, thus allowing faster passage to the main absorptive site, the small intestine. Diarrhoea hinders absorption because of the extreme speed of passage. Slow gastric emptying (e.g. in the presence of **atropine** or **morphine**) may increase the time taken for drugs to be absorbed. TTFFT

Passage of drugs from the bloodstream to extravascular tissues

1. like skeletal muscle occurs very slowly with drugs which are highly ionized at pH 7.4.
2. like brain can only take place if the substances are highly lipid-soluble.
3. or from extravascular tissues to the blood occurs with similar difficulty in whichever direction they move.
4. is generally insignificant for the molecules of drugs which are bound to plasma proteins.
5. is essential if drugs are to exert a biological effect.

Many of the factors which affect the passage of drugs from gut lumen to bloodstream apply to the further movement of drugs to the extravascular tissues and spaces. However, the endothelial cells of the capillaries are generally less tightly packed than others and the hydrostatic pressure drives fluid through the pores and through *intercellular spaces*, carrying with it free drug molecules. Larger molecules, like plasma proteins and any drug bound to them, will not cross the capillary wall with such ease. However, the equilibrium between bound and free drug molecules means that, as unbound drug leaves the plasma, other molecules are freed from their protein binding sites to preserve the equilibrium in the bloodstream. In this way drugs readily reach the tissues on which they act. A drug could act entirely within the bloodstream if, for example, it were an anticoagulant like **heparin**, or if the drug's effect was merely to displace another from its protein binding site.

For drugs to reach the CNS, a different barrier has to be crossed. The endothelial cells appear to be packed more closely together in the capillaries supplying the brain and spinal cord, so that, to reach the CNS, substances must pass through the endothelial *cells* rather than through the intercellular spaces. Therefore many electrolytes penetrate to the brain poorly or not at all, depending on their extent of ionization at plasma pH. Only the non-ionized drug is highly lipid-soluble, a property which is essential for most chemicals to diffuse rapidly across biological membranes.

Some parts of the brain capillary bed are more permeable than others to drugs, particularly in the hypothalamus and the area postrema. Drugs gaining access at these places can diffuse throughout the brain tissue, which is bathed in cerebrospinal fluid. However, the absorptive surface area is small and proportionally few drug molecules penetrate. Furthermore, the whole brain has a much larger volume than those regions into which absorption occurs so that distant parts of the CNS are likely to be exposed to low drug concentrations only.

It should be noted that the impediment to drug uptake into the brain is mirrored by equal difficulties for drugs to escape the brain back into the bloodstream. Neither the ionic composition nor the pH of the cerebrospinal fluid (pH 7.3) is markedly different from the corresponding values in plasma ultrafiltrate (though it is virtually cell- and protein-free). Therefore the degree of ionization of weak electrolytes will be similar to that in plasma. FFTTF

MCQ 7

The apparent volume of distribution of a drug in man

1. can exceed the volume of water in the body.
2. would be expected to be about 12 litres if the drug did not penetrate cells and remained in the circulation.
3. is unaffected by renal excretion.
4. will have a misleadingly low value if the drug is sequestered at extravascular sites.
5. can be calculated only if data are available on drug concentrations in extra- and intracellular water.

To minimize toxic hazards of drugs (particularly those with a low therapeutic index) when they are given to patients with serious renal, hepatic or cardiac impairment, it is important to know the distribution of the drugs. One measurement is the volume of distribution (V_d); this is the apparent volume of liquid in which the drug is distributed and can be calculated from drug concentrations in blood samples.

Suppose a drug is unable to penetrate cells and leaves the circulation very slowly (e.g. the highly protein-bound dye **Evan's Blue**). After a few minutes to allow for mixing, it would be distributed solely in the plasma (about 3 litres). This volume could be calculated from $V_d = Q/C$, where Q is the total amount of drug in the circulation (i.e. the dose, if given i.v.) and C is the concentration in plasma.

Some substances (e.g. **iodide** and sucrose) are distributed in the total extracellular fluid volume; that is, they penetrate cells very poorly but get into the extravascular space and interstitial water and would yield a V_d of about 12 litres. Finally, water itself or some very lipid-soluble materials which penetrate cells easily may become evenly distributed throughout total body water, though this may take an hour or more to occur. In such cases V_d would be about 40 litres – equivalent to about 60% of body weight.

Similar values can be measured for a variety of drugs but there are many pitfalls in interpretation. Suppose the *total* drug concentration in plasma was measured of a drug which was actually distributed throughout the extracellular fluid but which was also highly bound to plasma protein. The extra material retained in the plasma would lead to the calculation of a low V_d value, which would suggest a less extensive distribution than was actually the case. Alternatively, drugs which are accumulated at extravascular sites (e.g. **thiopentone** in fat) can be present in plasma in such low concentrations that an enormous V_d value can be calculated, perhaps exceeding the total available body water. Because they bind so avidly with tissues, the drugs **imipramine** (a tricyclic antidepressant) and **propranolol** (a β-adrenoceptor blocking drug) have V_d values greater than 1000 and 250 litres respectively, despite the fact that they both bind well to plasma proteins.

Finally, the rate of loss of a drug through biotransformation or excretion may be rapid enough to prevent a distribution plateau being reached after a single dose. Therefore V_d is calculated from a *theoretical* plasma concentration derived by extrapolating to zero time (when excretion and biotransformation will be zero) the relationship between plasma concentration and time after administration. TFFFF

Excretion of plasma-borne substances by the kidney

1. can be used to calculate renal blood flow.
2. can be expressed by renal clearance, which may exceed 600 ml min^{-1}.
3. involves active secretion if the clearance ratio (renal clearance to glomerular filtration rate) is greater than 1.0.
4. can only be related to eventual elimination of a substance if its apparent volume of distribution and other sites of loss are known.
5. will not normally occur if their molecular weight is greater than 1000 daltons.

Drugs and their metabolites are eventually eliminated from the body by excretion in sweat, exhaled air, bile, faeces and, most importantly, urine. About 25% of cardiac output flows through the kidneys and the short renal arteries take blood to the glomerular capillaries with little drop in pressure. Many blood-borne substances (even large polypeptides of molecular mass up to 65 000 daltons) appear in the glomerular filtrate but the larger proteins to which drugs bind do not. Many lipid-soluble drugs are reabsorbed from the lumen of the proximal tubule, but polar molecules remain in the lumen unless a carrier system exists for their reabsorption.

Renal excretion can be quantified by measuring the volume of urine produced in a particular time and the amount of drug in it. More usually the 'clearance' of a drug is calculated and can provide insight into the way the kidney handles the drug. Renal clearance (Cl_R), in millilitres per minute, represents the volume of plasma water from which the drug must be totally removed to provide the amount appearing in the urine in 1 min. $Cl_R = Q/C$, where Q is the amount of drug excreted per minute and C its concentration in the plasma.

Suppose a drug is not bound to plasma proteins, is freely filtered at the glomerulus but is neither secreted nor reabsorbed in the tubules. Its Cl_R would be equal to the glomerular filtration rate (GFR). Since the glomerulus filters about 20% of the blood delivered, the GFR is about 130 ml min^{-1}. For a substance normally totally reabsorbed by the tubules (e.g. glucose), $Cl_R = 0$. By contrast, **penicillin** is so rapidly *secreted* into the tubules that the renal arterial plasma is almost completely cleared in a single passage through the kidney. The Cl_R of such a molecule can provide information on renal blood flow: a value of about 650 ml min^{-1} means that total renal blood flow (plasma represents about 50% of blood volume) is some 1300 ml min^{-1} (i.e. about 25% of cardiac output).

The ratio of Cl_R to GFR is called the clearance ratio. A value of 1 suggests a drug is excreted by filtration alone, a ratio >1 implies some active secretion, and <1 some reabsorption.

To discover the extent to which plasma drug concentration is reduced by renal excretion, the apparent volume of distribution (V_d) is needed. The greater the value of V_d, the longer it will normally take for a drug to be eliminated. The elimination rate constant, K_{el}, is given by the plasma clearance rate, Cl_P, divided by the volume of distribution ($K_{el} = Cl_P/V_d$), but K_{el} represents the sum of rate constant values for all sites of loss. Only if a drug is excreted unchanged and solely by the kidneys will total plasma clearance equal renal clearance. TTTTF

MCQ 9

The half-life $(t_{1/2})$ of a drug in the plasma

1. is expressed as the percentage that remains half an hour after administration.
2. will be short if the drug gets into the enterohepatic circulation.
3. will have a higher value if a drug is distributed throughout the body water rather than the plasma water.
4. cannot be calculated if the drug is secreted into the bile.
5. is not a constant in an individual since the presence of other drugs can modify drug elimination.

The elimination of drugs through the kidney can be expressed mathematically through terms like renal clearance (Cl_R) and the apparent volume of distribution (V_d). If a drug is excreted unchanged and solely by the kidney, then its rate constant of elimination $K_{el} = Cl_R/V_d$. Since the half-life $(t_{1/2})$ of an exponential process is given by $0.693/K$, then $t_{1/2} = 0.693V_d/Cl_R$.

Suppose that three drugs A, B and C are distributed respectively in plasma water $(V_d = 3$ litres), extracellular water $(V_d = 12$ litres) and total body water $(V_d = 40$ litres). If each drug was eliminated solely by glomerular filtration with no reabsorption (glomerular filtration rate $= Cl_R = 130$ ml min.$^{-1}$), the half-lives would be: A, 16 min; B, 64 min; C, 213 min. By contrast, if each was eliminated by tubular secretion $(Cl_R = 650$ ml min^{-1}), the respective half-lives would be 3.2, 12.8 and 42.6 min. Quite obviously, no matter how large a clearance value, any drug with a large V_d value would be eliminated slowly. Thus the cardiac glycoside **digoxin**, 75% of which is eliminated by the kidneys, has a clearance of 130 ml min^{-1} but a V_d of 640 litres, so its half-life is about 42 h. **Frusemide**, a diuretic, is 66% eliminated in the urine and has a similar clearance (140 ml min^{-1}), but since its V_d is 8 litres its half-life is about 1.5 h.

Some drugs are removed from plasma by the liver and reach the intestinal lumen via the bile. If intestinal reabsorption then occurs, a drug may be recycled for long periods within the enterohepatic circulation. Gradually, biotransformation and urinary excretion may help remove such a drug from the body. Biliary excretion is important for some organic electrolytes that are not reabsorbed from the intestine because they are largely ionized at luminal pH (e.g. **bromosulphophthalein**, used in liver function tests). A specific active transport process appears to be responsible for the secretion of organic anions and cations into the bile since it occurs against a concentration gradient (bile to plasma concentration ratios can exceed 25 : 1) and competition between substances can occur for the transport. Thus the half-lives of drugs can be altered by the presence of others which affect their excretion.

Generally, polar compounds of molecular weight >400 daltons are favoured for biliary excretion. Many glucuronide conjugates of drugs (or more usually of drug metabolites) are secreted into the bile but most of them are recycled through the enterohepatic circulation because β-glucuronidase in the duodenum releases the previously conjugated chemical. FFTFT

The graph relates time after i.v. administration of 150 mg of a drug to the concentration (on a log₁₀ scale) of the drug in the plasma. It can be concluded that

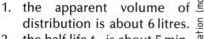

1. the apparent volume of distribution is about 6 litres.
2. the half-life $t_{1/2}$ is about 5 min.
3. the plasma clearance is about 150 ml min^{-1}.
4. if, between 15 and 25 min, 25 mg of drug was eliminated in urine, the renal clearance is 2.5 mg min^{-1}.
5. little biotransformation of the drug takes place.

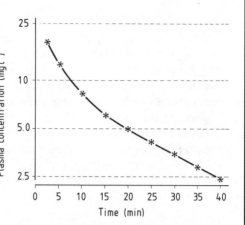

The apparent volume of distribution, V_d is the volume of water into which the dose (D) of a drug must be distributed to give the concentration appearing in the plasma. It is a proportionality constant which relates the amount of drug in the body at time t to the concentration in the plasma at that time (C_t). Thus $V_d = D/C_t$. The V_d must be calculated as if the drug had been given a moment earlier since only at this instant is the amount of the drug in the body known accurately; at any later time some may have been biotransformed or excreted. To obtain V_d, the value for C_t at time 0 is required (at which moment D was 150 mg) and can be found by extrapolating the linear part of the plasma concentration–time plot back to its intersection with the y-axis, giving a value of 10 mg l^{-1}. The plot deviates from linearity in the early time points because distribution and mixing of the drug are still taking place. The V_d is therefore 150/10 = 15 litres.

The $t_{1/2}$ is the time taken for the plasma concentration to be reduced by 50%. It takes 20 min for the concentration to fall from 5 to 2.5 mg l^{-1} and this is a good estimate of $t_{1/2}$; equally well the $t_{1/2}$ could be estimated from any other values on the linear part of the plot. The early non-linear portions should not be used in this calculation because distribution and mixing of the drug within the body are still taking place.

The linear part of the log₁₀ plasma concentration–time plot can be represented by the equation $C_t = C_0 e^{-kt}$, where C_0 and C_t are the initial plasma concentration and the concentration after time t respectively and k is the rate constant of elimination. The exponential term e can be removed from this equation by converting values to their natural logs (ln) and the equation may then be rewritten $\ln(C_t/C_0) = -kt$. From this equation the $t_{1/2}$ can be obtained as follows. When $C_t/C_0 = 1/2$ (i.e. sufficient time has passed for the plasma concentration to halve), $\ln(C_t/C_0) = \ln(1/2) = -kt$, where $t =$ the $t_{1/2}$. Rearranging, $t_{1/2} = \ln 2/k = 0.693/k$.

Plasma clearance (Cl_P) is the overall volume of plasma completely cleared of the drug in 1 min whether clearance is by excretion in the urine or bile or through biotransformation.

continued on next page 11

$$Cl_P = kV_d = \frac{0.693\ V_d}{t_{\frac{1}{2}}} = 0.522 \text{ litres min}^{-1}$$

Renal clearance represents the volume of plasma which must be cleared of drug to provide that amount of drug excreted in the urine. A total of 25 mg was excreted between 15 and 25 min, when the plasma concentration averaged (mid-point of the time interval) 5 mg l^{-1}. Renal clearance is therefore 0.5 litres min^{-1}. Note that units of clearance are volume per unit time.

If the rate at which the kidney clears the drug from the plasma (renal clearance) is the same as the overall rate at which the drug disappears from the plasma (plasma clearance), then biotransformation must be a very minor route for removal of the drug because renal excretion can wholly account for the loss of drug. FFFFT

The bioavailability of a drug

1. is defined as the ratio of the actual blood concentration attained to that required to produce a pharmacological effect after a particular dose has been given.
2. given by mouth must be 100% if the drug is completely absorbed.
3. will be unaffected by changes in formulation.
4. is a term applied only to oral administration.
5. may be affected by liver damage.

Bioavailability may be defined in two ways. In simple terms it is the fraction (or percentage) of an administered dose which reaches the systemic circulation. In these terms bioavailability is often less than 100% for drugs given p.o. since they may be destroyed in the gut, poorly absorbed, biotransformed in the liver or enter the enterohepatic circulation. For most drugs given i.v., bioavailability is 100%. This simple approach to bioavailability does not take into account the fact that a minimal plasma level is required for the drug to be effective. Thus, although 100% of a dose may eventually appear in the systemic circulation, absorption may be so slow that an effective plasma level is never reached. To think of this as being 100% bioavailability is unhelpful. Therefore *both* the rate at which a drug becomes available to the systemic circulation and the proportion of the dose which becomes available are often taken into account in a more sophisticated concept of bioavailability, though it is much more difficult to express this concept quantitatively.

Variations in drug formulation can bring about large changes in bioavailability whichever concept is used. If the active ingredients are set in a small ball of cement, bioavailability will be low (or zero). Suppose a drug is rapidly and completely absorbed from the gut and is excreted unchanged in the urine. A dose is given which permits the minimum effective concentration (MEC) in the blood to be reached in 1 h and maintained for 3 h, the peak level being double the MEC. Two new formulations are made, both of which slow absorption. With one the slowing is so great that the MEC is never reached and the drug is ineffective. Yet it is totally absorbed and on the simple definition its bioavailability would be 100%. The other formulation delays absorption and the MEC is not reached until 3 h after administration; blood levels are maintained slightly higher than the MEC for 2–3 h and the concentration then gradually falls to zero. The area under the curve for all three formulations (i.e. the proportion of the dose available to the systemic circulation) could be the same but the longest delayed biological effect of smallest intensity would generally be the least desirable. FFFFT

The dose

1. of a drug, if given infrequently, will result in lower but steadier plasma levels than the same dose given more frequently.
2. of any drug subject to a first pass effect can be raised so as to provide a higher concentration in the plasma.
3. and plasma concentration of a drug principally secreted in the bile should be monitored in patients with hepatic impairment.
4. schedule ideally should be constructed so as to provide a minimum effective drug concentration at all times during therapy.
5. of a drug largely removed by a first pass effect must be lower when given i.v. than p.o. in order to achieve the same peripheral plasma level.

It is most useful to think of bioavailability as involving both the *rate* at which and the *extent* to which an administered drug reaches the systemic circulation. Any drug given by mouth and absorbed from the stomach or small intestine might be biotransformed and/or excreted into the bile, so reducing the amount getting to the systemic circulation. The more a drug is affected by these hepatic processes, the lower will be its bioavailability after oral administration. A 'first pass effect' occurs when a large fraction of a drug is lost as it passes for the first time through the liver (i.e. in a high concentration in the portal blood). For drugs affected in this way it may be possible to achieve a minimum effective concentration (MEC) in blood by simply giving a larger dose p.o. since the fractional bioavailability will not be altered in most cases. With some drugs (e.g. **propranolol**), however, the fraction of an oral dose that gets to the systemic circulation does change with the size of the dose given, suggesting that the hepatic processes may have become saturated.

Drugs which are readily extracted by the liver will exhibit plasma levels which vary greatly from patient to patient. Impairment of hepatic function or blood flow may markedly increase the bioavailability of a drug subject to a prominent first pass effect.

It is desirable that drug administration should produce a fairly steady plasma level above the MEC but below the level at which toxicity is seen. Unless a drug has a long half-life and therefore needs to be given infrequently, there may be large fluctuations in plasma concentrations with successive administrations. This is often tolerable provided that the peaks do not reach toxic levels and the troughs do not fall below the MEC (however, the variation in the intensity of the biological effect might be unacceptable). With many drugs a compromise is necessary since steady levels will result if many small doses are given at frequent intervals – the ideal situation would be i.v. infusion – but in practice most drugs are given intermittently. With a drug whose MEC is $25\,\mu g\,ml^{-1}$ and with a clearance of $50\,ml\,min^{-1}$ it would be necessary to infuse $50 \times 25 = 1.25\,mg\,min^{-1}$ to maintain a steady-state concentration equal to the MEC. Intermittent dosing could be used giving, say, 150 mg every 2 h or 600 mg every 8 h but clearly the greater the interval between doses, the greater the fluctuations in plasma level. FTTTT

The biotransformation of chemical substances in the body

1. may increase pharmacological activity.
2. only applies to 'foreign' substances (xenobiotics).
3. requires a phase I reaction to be followed by a phase II reaction before a metabolite is produced.
4. usually involves a conversion to a less polar and hence more lipid-soluble material.
5. often enables rapid excretion of otherwise persistent drugs to take place.

The duration of action of a drug is usually dependent on the time for which an adequate concentration remains in the body, though there are exceptions. Some toxins, for example, produce structural damage to nerves from which recovery never occurs.

Many drugs are polar in nature, are readily excreted by the kidney and do not easily cross membranes, which may restrict their access to bio-transforming enzymes. Such drugs often undergo little biotransformation. However, most drugs are non-polar and are lipid-soluble. Their lipid solubility is the factor which reduces their renal excretion by permitting, first, a wider distribution of the drug in the body (and hence a lower concentration to be delivered to the kidney) and, second, reabsorption of the drug from the kidney tubules. Lipid solubility also gives the drug access to 'drug-metabolizing enzymes', which generally lie beyond several lipid membranes in the endoplasmic reticulum in the liver. Therefore, such drugs are often extensively biotransformed. The action of these enzymes is not confined to foreign compounds (xenobiotics) but extends to materials which occur naturally in the body or diet (e.g. steroids, bile acids). Indeed, it may have been in order to cope with naturally occurring materials that the drug-metabolizing enzymes evolved.

Enzymic conversion into more water-soluble products can greatly change the excretory pattern of a lipid-soluble drug. Some barbiturates (e.g. **thiopentone**) would remain in the body for several years if they were not biotransformed and then excreted. Biotransformation generally reduces pharmacological activity but there are many exceptions to this rule (e.g. the organophosphorus anticholinesterase **parathion** to **paraoxon**; **imipramine** to **desmethylimipramine**, which has equivalent or greater antidepressant activity). Substances which need to be chemically converted to produce their full pharmacological effect are called 'pro-drugs'. Whilst biotransformation helps eliminate many materials, some metabolic products may be carcinogenic, mutagenic or teratogenic.

Biotransformations are often divided into phase I, where a functional group such as $-NH_2$ or $-OH$ is introduced or created, and phase II, where highly polar conjugates like glucuronides are formed with the drug or its phase I metabolite. Not all drugs undergo both phases and either phase may produce a less active and more water-soluble (and therefore excretable) metabolite. TFFFT

MCQ 14

Phase I biotransformations occurring in the liver

1. usually involve the microsomal enzymes (e.g. mixed function oxidases).
2. may involve enzymes located on the smooth endoplasmic reticulum.
3. are carried out by enzymes which are highly specific for their substrates.
4. are controlled by a rate-limiting step involving the binding of drug to the scarce enzyme cytochrome P-450.
5. may conjugate drugs with glycine.

Enzymes capable of biotransforming drugs exist in many cells (and e.g. in plasma) but, for most drugs, biotransformation takes place in the liver. Its location and portal venous blood supply make the liver well suited to modifying chemical substances, especially those absorbed from the gut (the usual route for drug administration).

Most enzymes concerned with drug biotransformation, especially phase I reactions, are found on the intracellular membranes of the rough and the smooth endoplasmic reticulum. Subcellular fractionation can isolate these membranes, which may then form independent vesicles called microsomes. In the smooth microsomes are many of the enzymes responsible for phase I biotransformations – a major group being the mixed function oxidases. In general, reactions with this system require molecular oxygen (one atom becoming bonded to the substrate, the other appearing as water), a reducing agent (often nicotine adenine disphosphonucleotide (reduced); NADPH) and, typically, two enzymes, cytochrome P-450 and cytochrome P-450 reductase.

During the formation of hydroxylated products (e.g. of **4-hydroxypropranolol** from **propranolol**) the drug first combines with cytochrome P-450 in its oxidized (ferric, Fe^{3+}) form. Cytochrome P-450 reductase converts this to the ferrous (Fe^{2+}) form by transferring an electron donated by NADPH. A second electron from the same source reduces molecular oxygen, which attaches to the drug–cytochrome P-450 complex. Finally, the oxygen is shifted to the drug molecule, one atom being used to form the hydroxylated product and the other to form water.

A great variety of drugs are transformed in this way, indicating that the substrate specificity of the enzymes is low. This low specificity explains why many drugs are subject to a first pass effect in the liver. Their lipid solubility permits speedy absorption from the gut and they are quickly passed at high concentration to the liver in the portal blood. Rapid uptake into hepatocytes then presents the drug to the microsomal enzyme systems. The low specificity also means that many drugs will compete with each other for binding to cytochrome P-450, which occurs in great abundance in the liver. It is the cytochrome P-450 reductase which is less plentiful and this makes the conversion of the drug–cytochrome–Fe^{3+} complex to its Fe^{2+} form the rate-limiting step.

Conjugation with glycine is a phase II reaction. TTFFF

Phase II biotransformations

1. produce non-toxic conjugates which need not be excreted quickly.
2. may involve substances which do not participate in phase I reactions.
3. are exemplified by the glucuronidation of **morphine**.
4. do not involve liver microsomal enzymes.
5. may give rise to products which are less water-soluble than the parent drug.

Several types of phase I biotransformation, such as oxidations (producing ketones or introducing hydroxyl groups) or reductions (e.g. of nitro to $-NH_2$ or of carboxyl to either aldehyde or alcohol) produce polar materials which are readily excreted in the urine. Some products may be more active pharmacologically than the parent compound and some may in fact be less water-soluble. Many of these metabolites and some of the parent compounds undergo phase II reactions when they become conjugated to glucuronic acid, for example, which makes the product more polar, more water-soluble and generally more readily excreted in the urine.

Drug biotransformation may involve simultaneous and/or sequential reactions with different enzymes and the products may be further biotransformed and/or conjugated with different materials. Usually the chemical structure of any drug favours only a few of the pathways. Therefore, of the dozens of potential metabolites, significant quantities of only a few are actually formed.

The most common conjugate is glucuronic acid (derived from glucose). It can be combined with hydroxyl or carbonyl groups (*O*-glucuronides) and with amino or sulphydryl groups (*N*- or *S*-glucuronides) to form water-soluble polar products which are often actively *secreted* into the tubules as well as passing into the urine in the glomerular filtrate. **Morphine** and **diazepam** are largely excreted as glucuronides though they will probably have undergone *N*-dealkylation and deamination respectively in phase I reactions before conjugation takes place.

Other conjugation reactions produce ethereal sulphates (from phenols) or acetylated products (from aromatic primary amines such as sulphonamides). Ironically, acetylated sulphonamides may be less soluble than the parent drug and may produce renal damage if high concentrations crystallize in the kidney tubules. Finally, methylation may occur, particularly of endogenous catecholamines (adrenaline and noradrenaline).

Mixed function oxidases occur almost entirely in microsomes but phase II enzymes may occur free in cytosol (acetyltransferases, methyltransferases) or in mitochondria (glycine transferase) or microsomes (UDP glucuronidyl transferase).

Phase II reactions do not always *de*-toxify a drug. *N*-Acetylation of **isoniazid** gives a reactive product which contributes to the severe liver damage sometimes produced by this antitubercular drug. FTTFT

MCQ 16

Biotransformation of drugs may be influenced by

1. genetic factors, an example being the very slow hydrolysis of **succinylcholine** in some individuals.
2. age, an example being when premature babies, because of their poor ability to form glucuronides, are rapidly poisoned by some drugs.
3. cardiac disease which, by reducing liver blood flow, may prolong the half-life of **lignocaine**.
4. viral hepatitis, which causes the induction of liver microsomal enzymes, thereby accelerating the breakdown of **chlordiazepoxide**.
5. species differences, explaining why humans are less sensitive to **atropine** than are rabbits.

The biotransformation of a compound depends on its chemistry, route of administration, distribution, dose and many other factors. There are many major differences between species in the way a drug is biotransformed (e.g. a highly active esterase, absent in man, is present in the plasma of rabbits, and this enables them to eat deadly nightshade with impunity). This type of difference has major implications in drug testing.

Genetic differences within a species can have a major influence. The action of **succinylcholine** is normally brief because it is hydrolysed by plasma esterases but some patients have an abnormal enzyme, genetically determined, which disposes of the drug so slowly that paralysis may last for an hour rather than the usual few minutes. Environmental pollutants, like smoke in cities or from tobacco, contain agents which can induce liver microsomal enzymes to biotransform drugs (e.g. **pentazocine**) more quickly than usual.

With regard to age differences, babies do not have a fully developed drug-metabolizing system and glucuronide formation is particularly slow. **Chloramphenicol** accumulates dangerously, if not excreted as the glucuronide, and its toxic effects cause the 'grey baby' syndrome.

State of health can affect biotransformation. Some drugs are biotransformed almost entirely by the liver and are greatly affected by changes in the rate of liver blood flow. **Lignocaine** and **pentazocine** are said to have a 'flow-limited' metabolism and will persist in the body for a longer period of time if the blood flow to the liver is reduced (in cardiac disease or if there are obstructions in hepatic vessels). More frequently, biotransformation will be affected by liver dysfunction such as in cirrhosis, hepatitis or fatty degeneration. Minor tranquillizers like **chlordiazepoxide** may have a considerably increased half-life in patients with viral hepatitis; even normal doses may accumulate to such an extent that the patient becomes comatose. The half-life of **digoxin** is longer in patients exhibiting hypothyroidism and shorter in patients with hyperactivity of the thyroid gland. Finally, heavy-metal poisoning and porphyria impair the formation and functioning of many liver microsomal enzymes and result in decreased hepatic biotransformation of some drugs. TTTFF

Biotransformation may be affected by

1. **phenobarbitone**, which accelerates the glucuronidation of bilirubin.
2. **cimetidine** which, by inhibiting cytochrome P-450, potentiates the actions of **chlordiazepoxide**.
3. **phenobarbitone**, which reduces the anticoagulant effect of **warfarin** by inducing cytochrome P-450.
4. **proadifen** (SKF 525A), which blocks glucuronidyl transferase and is used clinically to minimize the first pass effect.
5. **secobarbitone**, which can reduce its own rate of biotransformation by formation of a reactive intermediate that irreversibly blocks cytochrome P-450.

The activity of enzymes involved in drug biotransformation can be increased or decreased by many substances. Especially when given repeatedly, drugs may induce the formation of microsomal enzymes by causing the enzyme to be synthesized faster than usual, possibly by interfering with a repressor substance which controls the rate at which messenger RNA is transcribed from DNA.

Cytochrome P-450 is the most commonly induced enzyme and exists in several isomeric forms which vary both in specificity and structure. One isoenzyme is induced by hydrocarbons in tobacco smoke, another by the medium- or long-term use of **phenobarbitone** (e.g. in epilepsy). **Phenobarbitone** is itself more quickly biotransformed (thus some tolerance develops), as are many other substances which are biotransformed by the same cytochrome P-450 (e.g. other barbiturates, coumarin anticoagulants and **chlorpromazine**). Thus a patient stabilized on **warfarin** and beginning a course of **phenobarbitone** would need to have the dose of **warfarin** increased to maintain the same prothrombin time.

Although as a rule enzyme induction is clinically undesirable, some attempts have been made to exploit it therapeutically. A genetic disorder causing decreased glucuronide formation leads to elevated bilirubin levels and patients appear jaundiced. **Phenobarbitone** induces glucuronidyl transferase (which conjugates bilirubin and thus enhances its excretion) and it may be possible to use low doses of **phenobarbitone** chronically to produce induction and alleviate the condition.

Some drugs inhibit biotransformation, especially if they are very lipid-soluble and remain dissolved in lipid membranes close to the microsomal enzymes. Others produce inhibition by competition with cytochrome P-450; **cimetidine** potentiates the actions of anticoagulants and of **chlordiazepoxide** by this mechanism. Reactive intermediates formed from some drugs (**spironolactone, secobarbitone, propylthiouracil**) may cause irreversible inhibition by covalent binding to cytochrome P-450.

Proadifen (SKF 525A) is a seemingly competitive inhibitor of biotransformation and is commonly used in laboratory studies but has no clinical use. It has a high affinity for cytochrome P-450 and can slow the phase I biotransformation of many substances. (It will prolong the 'sleeping time' of mice given, say, **hexobarbitone**.) Its effect rapidly decreases even if repeated doses are given. TTTFT

Drug Actions, Interactions and Receptors

In the measurement of drug action

1. an acute toxicity test in rodents will provide quantal data.
2. the safety margin is indicated by the therapeutic index, which can be estimated as the ratio $ED_{50} : LD_{50}$.
3. all-or-none events must be analysed by binary mathematics.
4. a therapeutic index in man is the ratio of the dose causing toxic effects to that causing beneficial effects.
5. the concentration calculated to produce a half-maximal response (EC_{50}) is a quantal measurement.

Biological responses produced by drugs are treated mathematically in different ways, depending on whether they are quantal or continuous (graded) responses. A quantal response is all-or-none; that is, an effect will occur or fail to occur. For example, **insulin** can cause convulsions in mice; either a convulsion occurs or it does not; a fraction of a convulsion cannot occur. In a *group* of mice, each given a particular dose of **insulin**, some will convulse and some will not. The proportion of convulsing mice in each group can be determined at various dose levels of **insulin** and then plotted graphically against the $\log_{10}$ of the doses. From this dose–response curve the ED_{50} value can be found. This is the dose calculated to be effective in 50% of the animals receiving it. The fewer the animals used in such experiments, the greater the uncertainty in the result. By the same token, measurements of desirable drug effects (e.g. the ability of hypnotic drugs to cause sleep or of antihistamines to counteract the lethal effect of injected **histamine**) can be analysed. In each case the ED_{50} values will be more prone to error the fewer the animals used.

Acute toxicity tests also yield quantal data, animals being either killed or not killed by a particular drug dose. A graph relating the proportion of a group dying to the dose given would now yield an LD_{50} (median lethal dose).

The $LD_{50} : ED_{50}$ ratio is called the therapeutic index and gives an indication of the safety margin of the drug. The higher the index, the better. Measurements of LD_{50} cannot, of course, be made in man (because of the shortage of volunteers), so the ratio between the doses producing toxic and beneficial effects is used clinically as a therapeutic index.

Note that ED_{50} (or EC_{50}) is sometimes used in a different context in relation to *continuous* responses, where it represents the dose (or concentration) required to produce a half-maximal response. TFFTF

MCQ 19

An example of a continuous (graded) response is

1. the degree of tachycardia induced by a cardiotonic drug in an anaesthetized dog.
2. the total extinction by a local anaesthetic of an action potential in a stimulated nerve.
3. the effect of a competitive neuromuscular blocking drug on the contraction of a single mammalian skeletal muscle fibre.
4. a drug-induced alteration in the volume of salivary secretion from an anaesthetized cat.
5. the degree of alteration in firing rate of spontaneously active central neurones by an iontophoretically applied drug.

An example of a quantal response is the production of convulsions by **insulin** in mice (a convulsion occurs or does not). However, the action of **insulin** can also be assessed as a continuous response by measuring how great a reduction it causes in the blood sugar level, which can be graded between zero and a maximal value. If the observer chooses to record those mice which show a fall in blood sugar of more than, say, 25% as 'responders' and those which show smaller falls as 'non-responders', then these continuous data will have been converted to a quantal form. The two types of response are, therefore, to some extent created by the observer. With both types of response the effect (however quantitated) is plotted against log dose and the dose–effect relationship determined; the more animals which contribute to the results, the more certainly will the relationship correspond to the true relationship between dose and response in that species and strain of animal.

Most types of pharmacological experiments use continuous response measurements (e.g. whenever the *magnitude* of a parameter is being monitored, like rate of neuronal firing, tension in a muscle or level of blood pressure) and they are usually more informative than those providing quantal data.

Dose–response curves for quantal and continuous responses often use an arithmetic scale on the y-axis (e.g. percentage maximum response) and a log_{10} scale on the x-axis. With quantal data, however, a more linear relationship is found if probit values are used instead of percentages of animals responding. The probit transformation expresses the percentage of animals responding in terms of standard deviations. Thus, if 66% of animals respond, the value would be 1 since 66% of observations in a normal distribution fall between +1 and −1 standard deviation. To eliminate negative values, 5 is added to each calculated value. Thus in the above example the probit value is 6. Values for all percentage responses can be found in published tables. This makes for a better linear relationship between log_{10} dose and response (now measured in probits) and easier comparison of two lines (e.g. in comparing toxicity data for two drugs). TFFTT

Drug receptors

1. are cell membrane components which initiate all pharmacological effects.
2. have complementary three-dimensional shapes to drugs and may interact preferentially with one stereoisomeric form of a drug.
3. are responsible for the selectivity in drug antagonism, such as occurs between **atropine** and **acetylcholine**.
4. when combining with an antagonist do not trigger a response.
5. can be separated intact from the remainder of the cell.

Most receptors are components of cell membranes and are capable of moving in the membrane and adapting in shape and distribution of charge when combined with a drug. Some receptors may move relatively large distances, being soluble cytoplasmic proteins which can bind drugs and then transport them to sites such as the cell nucleus. All receptors can combine with complementary agonistic drugs to form a complex that may trigger a biological response. Antagonists also bind to receptors but are unable to trigger a response. In the presence of an antagonist, agonists are less effective. The interactions between mixtures of drugs acting at the same receptors can be expressed and analysed mathematically.

Several lines of evidence suggest the existence of receptors:

(a) Highly selective antagonists exist (e.g. **histamine**, **acetylcholine** and **barium** cause guinea-pig ileum to contract but **mepyramine** in low concentration antagonizes only **histamine**).
(b) Stereoisomers, despite being physicochemically similar, are often dramatically different in potency.
(c) Not all cells respond equally. Some may contain no receptors for a given drug and therefore will not respond.
(d) Minor chemical changes, especially when they cause alteration to the molecular shape, may considerably influence drug activity.
(e) Drugs bind to minute membrane fragments and intact cells in similar rank order of effectiveness. This property may be retained when the fragments are inserted into artificial membranes. Further, recombinant DNA technology permits the synthesis of polypeptides with identical amino acid sequences to those in receptors and which bind drugs similarly.

Not all pharmacological effects are thought to involve cellular receptors. For instance, anaesthetics depress neuronal firing without having to bind to complementary sites in the membranes; bulk purgatives increase faecal volume and stimulate peristalsis without such binding. FTTTT

Drug-receptor interactions

1. are usually analysed on the assumption that the law of mass action is obeyed.
2. are affected by the concentration of the drug applied.
3. can be mathematically analysed only when experiments are done *in vitro*.
4. may be analysed to yield affinity constants, which for a particular drug is a constant value irrespective of the tissue on which the drug acts.
5. may be characterized by affinity constants whose units are litres per mole.

Interactions between drugs and their receptors are assumed to obey the law of mass action and many predictions based on this assumption can be shown to be correct. Thus responses to drugs are dose-dependent, two different drugs can compete with each other for a common site of action and drug-receptor interactions can be treated quantitatively.

There are three major factors which determine the magnitude of the response to a drug: first, the number of drug molecules present (expressed as molar concentration); second, the proportion of available receptors occupied by the drug; third, the rate at which drug-receptor complexes are formed and/or broken.

Drug-receptor interactions can be expressed mathematically. Let $[D]$ be the molar concentration of the drug, r the proportion of receptors occupied in forming complexes and k_1 and k_2 association and dissociation rate constants respectively. Then at equilibrium the rates of formation and breakdown will be equal (or there would be no equilibrium) and so

$$k_1[D](1-r)=k_2r \quad \text{or} \quad (k_1/k_2)[D]=r/(1-r)$$

The ratio k_1/k_2 is the affinity constant (K_D; measured in litres per mole).

Enzyme kinetics can be expressed similarly and a ratio of rate constants, k_2/k_1 in the above equation, is the Michaelis-Menten constant, which is a dissociation constant (the reciprocal of affinity constant) with units of moles per litre.

From the equation $K_D[D]=r/(1-r)$, derived from the equilibrium condition, it can be seen that a simple reciprocal relationship exists between the affinity constant of a drug and the concentration needed to occupy 50% of the receptors (i.e. $K_D=1/[D]$, because at this degree of occupation $r=0.5$ and therefore $(1-r)=0.5$, so that $K_D[D]=1$).

Knowledge of affinity constants of drugs (especially antagonists) can be used to test if receptors in different tissues are identical (the affinity constant of a drug is then identical in the different tissues). Also, the selectivity of antagonists can be compared and drug concentrations required to produce chosen degrees of receptor blockade can be calculated if the appropriate affinity constants are known. TTFFT

In experiments to determine the affinity constant (K₁) of an antagonist

1. for a particular receptor the value will vary for each agonist against which it is measured.
2. it is necessary that receptors combine one-to-one with drug molecules, whether agonists or antagonists.
3. more than one concentration of antagonist must be used.
4. it is assumed that an agonist always occupies the same fraction of available receptors when it produces identically sized responses.
5. it is feasible to use a single agonist concentration throughout the experiment.

There are many assumptions made and several sources of error in determining the affinity constant of an antagonist.

Equations can be derived which relate the degree of occupation of the receptors (r) to the affinity constant and to the concentrations of *both* agonist (D) and antagonist (I) when they are present simultaneously and have reached equilibrium in competing for the same receptors; for example:

$$r = \frac{K_D[D]}{1 + K_D[D] + K_I[I]}$$

where K_D and K_I are affinity constants and [D] and [I] are molar concentrations of agonist and antagonist respectively.

It is assumed that drug D occupies exactly the same proportion of receptors (r) whenever it causes the same-sized response (irrespective of whether antagonist is present or not). The concentration of drug D required to occupy fraction r will vary according to the amount of competing drug, so a similar equation can be constructed for each concentration of the two drugs. From these relationships (r being of equal value) comes the so-called 'null equation':

$$K_I = \frac{\text{agonist 'dose ratio'} - 1}{\text{antagonist molar concentration}} = \frac{([D']/[D]) - 1}{[I]}$$

where [D'] is the concentration of drug D needed in the presence of [I] to produce a response equal in size to that produced by [D] in the absence of inhibitor. In each case the same fractional occupation (r) has been assumed to occur.

[D']/[D] can be seen to be a 'dose ratio'. Thus the affinity constant of an antagonist can be calculated from data which are readily measured and accumulated. Although experiments may be designed which offer more substantial data and make fewer assumptions than others, the minimum requirement is that a dose ratio is obtained for an agonist in the presence of an inhibitor. FTFTF

MCQ 23

The affinity constant (K_I) of an antagonist

1. equals the reciprocal of that antagonist concentration which reduces by half the size of the response to a given agonist dose.
2. can only be determined accurately at equilibrium, even if 60 min or more is required for equilibrium to be achieved.
3. is also known as the pA_2 value.
4. will be a larger numerical value the more potent the antagonist.
5. can be calculated from shifts of agonist concentration–response curves determined in the presence of different antagonist concentrations.

Determinations of the affinity constant (K_I) of an antagonist are based on measurements of an agonist dose ratio in the presence of that antagonist. An experiment might begin by obtaining reproducible responses of about half-maximal size to an agonist drug D. Next, by trial and error, and in the continuing presence of a fixed concentration of antagonist I, another dose of drug D could be found that caused a response matching the previous one. The affinity constant could then be calculated from the so-called 'null equation':

$$K_I = \frac{\text{agonist 'dose ratio'} - 1}{\text{antagonist molar concentration}}$$

Alternatively, the *antagonist* concentration could be altered over a narrow range in an attempt to find a concentration in the presence of which the agonist dose must be doubled to match its control response. In this situation the 'dose ratio' would be 2 (i.e. a doubling of the agonist concentration in the presence of I has produced an identical response to the control) and K_I would be equal to the reciprocal of the molar concentration of the antagonist present [I].

In the most common experimental design, complete concentration–response curves are determined for the agonist, first in the absence and then in the presence of known concentrations of the antagonist. A displacement to the right of the original curve will occur; the horizontal separation of successive curves provides the dose ratio values. Using the 'null equation' shown above, the antagonist affinity constant can then be calculated.

Early estimates of antagonist potency utilized 'pA_x', where x was most often 2 (i.e. pA_2, defined as the negative log of the molar concentration of antagonist required so that the dose of agonist must be doubled to maintain the same response). Since, with a dose ratio of 2, $K_I = 1/[I]$ and by definition $pA_2 = -\log_{10}[I]$, then $pA_2 = \log K_I$.

Many assumptions are made in these experiments:

(a) that the drug concentrations in the bath are identical to those surrounding the receptors;
(b) that the receptors are on the external surface of the membrane and each binds with just one drug molecule at a time;
(c) that drugs are in equilibrium with their receptors and are not metabolized or removed by the tissue.
(d) that short-term regulatory changes affecting receptor numbers do not occur.

Steps are often taken in experiments to minimize drug losses, for example by blocking tissue uptake of noradrenaline or by inhibiting enzymatic breakdown of acetylcholine. FTFTT

Drug antagonism

1. cannot occur unless substances act on the same type of receptor.
2. is of the functional type when the antagonist decreases the effect of a neuro-transmitter on an organ or tissue.
3. is competitive when a 1000-fold increase in dose is required for a drug to inhibit the response to a different agonist.
4. can be expressed by pA_x, the pA_{10} having a higher numerical value than the pA_2 for a competitive antagonist.
5. is competitive when an Arunlakshana–Schild plot is a straight line.

A pA_2 value can be calculated for any drug which reduces the effect of another. (pA_2 is defined as the negative log of the molar concentration of antagonist required so that the concentration of agonist must be doubled to maintain the same response.) However, the calculation is only meaningful for drugs which compete for the same receptor since pA_2 is related to the affinity constant (K_I) of an antagonist for its receptor.

If a drug reduces to the same extent the responses of a tissue to at least three agonists which act on different receptors, then it is likely to be a *functional* antagonist. If the drug is highly selective against only one type of agonist, then interaction at a common receptor is likely. Deductions about the type of antagonism are best made from $\log_{10}$ dose–response curves to agonists determined in the presence and absence of antagonists. The 'null equation' for a competitive antagonist, I, is

$$K_I = \frac{\text{agonist 'dose ratio'} - 1}{\text{antagonist molar concentration}}$$

which rearranges to

$$\text{dose ratio} = 1 + K_I[I]$$

This equation applies to all values of receptor occupation (i.e. for any size of biological response). Thus $\log_{10}$ dose–response curves to an agonist should be entirely parallel and shifted proportionally to the right as the concentration of antagonist is increased. If the curves are not parallel, the antagonism is not competitive.

From a family of agonist dose–response curves obtained in the presence of different concentrations of antagonist, it is possible to tabulate dose ratios corresponding to each antagonist concentration for graphical analysis as follows.

Using the relationship $pA_2 = \log_{10}K_I$, the equations above may be rearranged to

$$\log_{10}(\text{dose ratio} - 1) = \log_{10}[I] + pA_2$$

an equation which is in the form $y = mx + c$. If $\log_{10}$ (dose ratio – 1) is plotted against $\log_{10}[I]$ (an Arunlakshana–Schild plot), a straight line will be obtained with the y-axis intercept equal to the pA_2. Since m has no counter-part in the above equation, the slope of the line will be unity. The intercept on the x-axis will be the negative pA_2 and may be a better way to obtain a pA_2 since the distance of extrapolation from experimental points will be less. These conditions will only be fulfilled if the antagonism is competitive and this forms a very rigorous test for the competitive nature of the antagonism. FFFFF

MCQ 25

Heart rate and mean blood pressure of each of 12 rats were measured before and after administration of a drug. In each animal the second measurements were lower by at least 10%.

1. Student's *t*-test may show there is no statistically significant difference between the means of the blood pressure measurements on the first and second occasions.
2. A paired *t*-test may show no statistically significant difference between the two sets of blood pressure readings.
3. If in Student's *t*-test a *P* value of 0.01 is obtained, it suggests that there is a 1 in 100 chance of the drug producing the effects seen.
4. A plot of fall in blood pressure against fall in heart rate has a correlation coefficient of 0.99, suggesting that the fall in heart rate caused the fall in blood pressure.
5. Non-parametric tests would be invalid if applied to this purely numerical data.

The *t*-test devised by Student (a pseudonym for William S. Gossett) examines the difference between two means in relationship to the spread of the individual values about these means. The calculations give the likelihood of the observed difference between means occurring by chance. In the above experiment, if the spread of the values of resting blood pressure is very wide, a simple *t*-test may show that the means are not statistically significantly different despite each reading on the first occasion being larger than the second.

A paired *t*-test examines the size of the *differences* between *pairs* of readings. If there is no significant change, then these differences will be small, some positive, others negative. This test is not affected by the spread of the initial values and is a better test to use in these circumstances.

From statistical tables a *t*-value will be found to have a corresponding *P*-value. A *P* of 0.01 indicates that there is a 1 in 100 likelihood of the observed difference being due to chance alone. Then the means are said to be statistically different. By convention, a $P < 0.05$ (i.e. 1 in 20 or 5%) is taken as the dividing line for statistical significance. This does not imply the difference is necessarily due to the drug treatment. The use of a control group could establish that the effect was due to the drug administered and not due to, say, the passage of time. It is important to distinguish between *statistically* significant and *clinically* significant. A change in plasma protein binding of a drug from 15% to 10% may be statistically significant but clinically irrelevant.

A correlation coefficient of 0.99 shows that the two effects are related in magnitude but gives no indication of any relationship between cause and effect. Both effects could be independent and unrelated to the use of the drug.

Non-parametric tests determine statistical significance based on order within a group or on sign. They make no allowance for the size of a difference. They make no assumptions about the distribution of the data (*t*-tests are only valid if the data points are normally distributed). A sign test on the differences would show a statistically significant effect. TFFFF

Adverse reactions to drugs may be

1. allergic, in which case prior exposure to the drug or a closely related substance must have taken place.
2. idiosyncratic, in which case prior exposure to the drug or a closely related substance need not have occurred.
3. toxic, in which case a larger than normal dose must have been taken.
4. anaphylactic, which means that a normally protective factor is missing.
5. tachyphylactic, which involves a fast developing skin eruption.

Adverse reactions can be classified in several ways. Toxic reactions of types normally seen after drug overdose may occur in some individuals after a normal dose. This increased susceptibility may be explained by interactions with concurrently administered drugs, by disease states or by pharmacokinetic or physiological differences between individuals. For instance, tinnitus is a normal response to excessive **aspirin** but may be experienced by some after 900 mg (a normal therapeutic dose).

Idiosyncratic reactions do not involve prior exposure to the drug and depend on the particular genetic constitution of the individual. If 900 mg of **aspirin** causes detachment of external auditory meatus (the patient's ears fall off), an idiosyncratic reaction has occurred. One problem in drug testing is the detection and prediction of idiosyncrasy. Even if only 1 in 20 000 show a particular idiosyncrasy, then out of 10 million who take the drug some 500 will be affected. Such a number occurring in the UK would be easily detected but, if the 500 were distributed worldwide, the idiosyncrasy might go undetected for longer.

Allergic responses require prior exposure to a drug or related material so that antibodies can be formed. Exposure may be non-medical and appreciable quantities of a drug may occur in the general environment (on dust or in milk; e.g. **penicillin**). In the anaphylactic type of reaction the antibody is reaginic (IgE) and, typically, fixed to mast cells. Reaction with antigen produces mast-cell degranulation, releasing histamine and heparin and activating enzymes involved in synthesis of kinins and eicosanoids. This type of reaction may be mild, affecting say the skin, or may be systemic and fatal (e.g. as may occur with **penicillin**). Other allergic reactions involve different types of antibody (IgG) or lymphocytes (T-cells). The reactions may be immediate or delayed, and may produce a variety of cellular consequences, including cytotoxicity.

Tachyphylaxis is not a term applied to adverse drug reactions. It describes a quickly developing tolerance to a drug effect. TTFFF

MCQ 27

Undesirable consequences may occur if monoamine oxidase inhibitors are administered concurrently with

1. **pethidine.**
2. thiazide diuretics.
3. **levodopa.**
4. local anaesthetics with **adrenaline** as a vasoconstrictor.
5. hypoglycaemic agents like **chlorpropamide.**

Monoamine oxidase (MAO) exists in two major isomeric forms called MAO-A and MAO-B, with differing substrate specificities and for which selective inhibitors are known. For instance, **clorgyline** preferentially inhibits MAO-A, **selegiline** MAO-B, while **phenelzine** lacks selectivity. Narcotic analgesics (e.g. **morphine**) are slightly potentiated by monoamine oxidase inhibitors (MAOIs) but the effect is of little clinical significance. With **pethidine**, however, a potentially fatal interaction may occur though not in all patients. Agitation, tremor, hyperpyrexia, coma, cardiovascular collapse and respiratory depression all may result but the cause of the syndrome is unclear. The syndrome can be treated with **chlorpromazine** or with **prednisolone.**

Thiazide diuretics (e.g. **chlorothiazide**) increase the loss of sodium, potassium and water and are also mild antihypertensive agents. Some MAOIs are also used as antihypertensive agents (**phenelzine**) though their main use is in the treatment of depression. The antihypertensive effects of the thiazides may therefore be potentiated. However, this is not a harmful interaction but is made use of clinically when the two agents are given in combination to some patients with high blood pressure.

Monoamine oxidase inhibitors interact with indirectly acting sympatho-mimetics (e.g. **tyramine** in cheese). Inhibition of MAO permits more unchanged amine to be absorbed from the gastrointestinal tract and less is deaminated in organs like the liver. Inhibition of MAO may also result in larger than normal noradrenaline stores in nerve terminals.

Levodopa is used in the therapy of Parkinson's disease, producing its beneficial action when biotransformed to dopamine. Only that fraction of **levodopa** which is accumulated in CNS neurones (such as the dopaminergic nerves of the nigrostriatal pathway) can contribute to the antiparkinsonian effect. Any additional dopamine which is produced from **levodopa** in the periphery may cause sympathomimetic effects and these are likely to be exaggerated in the presence of MAOIs. Thus a hypertensive crisis (α_1-adrenoceptor stimulation in arterioles) sometimes accompanied by cardiac dysrhythmias (β_1-adrenoceptor stimulation) may be provoked if, for example, **phenelzine** is given concurrently. The MAO-B inhibitor **selegiline** is presently being used in combination with a reduced dose of **levodopa** to treat parkinsonism since it potentiates only central dopamine. Thus even potentially dangerous foods containing **tyramine** may be safely eaten. No clinically relevant interaction takes place with locally injected **adrenaline**, whose action is usually terminated by redistribution and uptake into cells.

The effects of hypoglycaemic agents (**insulin** and the oral hypoglycaemic drugs such as **tolbutamide** and **chlorpropamide**) are enhanced by MAOIs and a reduction by as much as 30% in **insulin** requirement may be seen. The mechanism is unclear but, since catecholamines affect blood sugar directly and modify insulin release, some interaction is possible. TFTFT

Undesirable interactions of clinical significance are likely to take place between

1. sulphonamides and **streptomycin**.
2. tetracyclines and antacids.
3. **aspirin** and antihistamines.
4. **streptomycin** and **pancuronium**.
5. **digitalis** and **spironolactone**.

Interactions between antibacterial drugs rarely lead to a reduction in the antibacterial effect but cases have been reported where bactericidal drugs such as **penicillin** show a reduced antibacterial effect when combined with bacteriostatic drugs (e.g. tetracyclines or **erythromycin**). Such combinations are best avoided. Useful interactions involving potentiation of the antibacterial effect are seen with the combination of a sulphonamide, **sulphamethoxazole**, and **trimethoprim** (**Co-trimoxazole**).

The antibacterial effect of tetracyclines is reduced when given with foods (e.g. milk) or with drugs containing large amounts of calcium, magnesium, aluminium or iron. Antacid preparations frequently contain (a) **calcium hydroxide** or **carbonate**; (b) **magnesium oxide**, **hydroxide**, **carbonate** or **trisilicate**; or (c) **aluminium hydroxide**. The tetracycline forms an insoluble complex with the metal ion and fails to be absorbed from the gastrointestinal tract. It is interesting to note that tetracyclines are not given to children under 7 years of age as the drugs complex with calcium in bones and teeth, producing a permanent yellow discolouration.

Aspirin, a non-steroidal anti-inflammatory drug, has additional analgesic and antipyretic effects. It is most frequently self-prescribed for headaches, rheumatic pains and to combat feverish episodes associated with virus infections. Antihistamines are used in minor allergic disorders like hay fever or skin rashes, but with few exceptions are sedative and may therefore cause drowsiness. There are no reported primary or secondary interactions between **aspirin** and antihistamines.

Streptomycin, in addition to its antibacterial actions, also has a stabilizing effect at the junction between the motor nerve and skeletal muscle. **Neomycin** and other aminoglycoside antibacterials act similarly. These drugs will therefore potentiate the effects of **tubocurarine** and other competitive neuromuscular blocking agents such as **pancuronium**.

Digitalis does interact with many potent diuretics (e.g. thiazides and frusemide) and with other agents which produce a hypokalaemia (e.g. glucocorticoids). The mechanism is controversial but the toxic effect of **digitalis** may be due to its inhibition of (Na^+, K^+)-ATPase. The further changes in plasma potassium exacerbate the ionic imbalance caused by this action. The effect is an important one as the margin between a toxic and effective dose of **digitalis** is small and any potentiation of the toxic effects is therefore serious. Potassium supplements can be given (**Slow-K**) or a potassium-sparing diuretic (**spironolactone** or **amiloride**) can be used in conjunction with therapy with **frusemide** or thiazides. FTFTF

MCQ 29

Clinically significant interactions are likely to take place between

1. tetracyclines and **warfarin** due to displacement from plasma protein binding.
2. sulphonamides and **tolbutamide** due to displacement from plasma protein binding.
3. **amitriptyline** and local anaesthetic solutions containing **adrenaline**.
4. barbiturates and **warfarin** due to the inhibition of liver microsomal enzymes.
5. **lincomycin** and **kaolin** due to changes in the pH of the gastrointestinal tract contents.

Although **warfarin** is highly bound to plasma albumin (95–98%), tetracyclines do not modify this binding significantly. However, they do increase the anticoagulant effect of **warfarin**. The mechanism is as follows. Gut flora are responsible for the synthesis of some 75% of the vitamin K available to the body (the remainder coming directly from the diet). The flora will be disturbed by tetracyclines, thereby lowering the availability of vitamin K. Since the action of **warfarin** in reducing the synthesis of clotting factors is mediated by an antagonism of vitamin K, the anticoagulant effect is increased. Although this effect is small in size, it is clinically significant because the prothrombin time (measure of blood coagulability) will have been carefully adjusted to an appropriate value in each patient before administration of the antibacterial drug.

Sulphonamides may be up to 95% bound (**sulphasalazine**) or only 60% bound (**sulphadiazine**). The oral hypoglycaemic agent **tolbutamide** is 95% bound and is displaced from its binding sites on albumin by sulpha drugs. If the binding were reduced from 95% to 90%, it should produce a doubling of the concentration of free drug but redistribution and excretion may counteract this tendency towards higher plasma levels. In many cases where an enhanced hypoglycaemia has occurred in the presence of sulphonamides, an inhibition of **tolbutamide** biotransformation has been postulated. Although there is no clear evidence to implicate displacement from plasma proteins in such episodes, simultaneous administration of these two groups of drugs should be undertaken cautiously.

Adrenaline (and **noradrenaline**) in local anaesthetic solutions is removed from the site of administration by blood flow and by active uptake into the noradrenergic nerves. **Amitriptyline** is a tricyclic antidepressant which blocks this uptake process, thus potentiating the local vasoconstriction and increasing the risk of cardiac dysrhythmias from the effects of **adrenaline** on the heart. In patients taking tricyclic antidepressants, 'plain' local anaesthetic solutions should be used or those formulated with **felypressin**.

Barbiturates generally, but **phenobarbitone** in particular, induce the formation of liver microsomal enzymes, which are responsible for the biotransformation of many drugs. The oral anticoagulant **warfarin** is affected and a small change in biotransformation may produce a large change in the dose needed to maintain a particular prothrombin time.

Kaolin (aluminium silicate) does not change the pH in the gastrointestinal tract but is highly effective in adsorbing some drugs – **lincomycin** and **promazine** in particular – thus reducing their absorption into the systemic circulation. FFTFF

Local Anaesthetics

MCQ 30

Under physiological conditions in a nerve at rest

1. the sodium ion concentration is greater in the intracellular than extracellular fluid.
2. a potential difference of about 70 mV occurs across the axonal membrane, the inside being negative with respect to the outside of the cell.
3. a metabolically active membrane pump expels chloride ions from inside the cell.
4. proteins within the cell provide a major contribution to the non-diffusible anions.
5. the axonal membrane is more permeable to potassium ions than to sodium ions.

In excitable cells (e.g. muscle and nerve) ions are distributed unequally between the intracellular and extracellular fluids (ICF and ECF). The ions Cl^- and K^+ diffuse relatively easily across the nerve membrane but this membrane is impermeable to large anions like proteins. The membrane is less permeable to Na^+ than to K^+ and a metabolically active pump expels Na^+ from the cell (in exchange for K^+). This selective permeability and the pump together account for the ion concentrations, which are: Na^+, about 150 mM ECF and 12 mM ICF; K^+, about 5 mM ECF and 150 mM ICF. Since the bulk of each fluid compartment is electrically neutral, the total positive charges are balanced by anions, principally the freely diffusible Cl^- and HCO_3^- in the ECF, whilst a much greater contribution to the ICF anion concentration comes from proteins and phosphates.

An electrical potential difference can be measured across the membrane of the cell, the inside being negative with respect to the outside. This potential is a consequence of the uneven distribution of the ions (particularly Cl^- and K^+) and their freedom to pass through the membrane. The K^+, present in a high concentration in the ICF, attempts to move down its concentration gradient, so producing a small excess in the immediate neighbourhood of the membrane outside the cell. Similarly, a few Cl^- ions accumulate adjacent to the membrane on the interior. This destroys electrical neutrality and leads to a build-up of opposite electrical charges on each side of the membrane, the effect of which is to halt the tendency of the ions to move down their concentration gradients since they now have to move against an electrical potential. Thus the membrane potential is established and the process reaches an equilibrium with 60–70 mV across the membrane, the inside being negative with respect to the outside. FTFTT

An action potential in a nerve fibre

1. is generated by a sudden inrush of sodium ions from the extracellular fluid.
2. will have a greater conduction velocity the smaller the fibre diameter.
3. is more slowly conducted if the fibre is myelinated because of the extra barrier to ionic movements.
4. decays because the membrane pump expels accumulating cations from the cell.
5. may measure in excess of 100 mV even though the resting potential of the membrane is only 60–70 mV.

A nerve impulse is detected as an electrical change conducted along the length of an axon (the action potential; AP). It involves a transient reversal of the membrane potential from the resting level of -70 mV to about $+40$ mV, brought about by a temporary but large increase in membrane permeability to Na^+.

The rising phase of the AP is caused by an inrush of Na^+ from the extracellular fluid (ECF) through channels in the membrane. This inrush is so rapid that it exceeds the capacity of the membrane pump to expel Na^+. Therefore these ions accumulate near the inside of the membrane and the intracellular fluid (ICF) becomes positively charged with respect to the ECF. As the AP continues to rise, K^+ begins to leave the ICF through channels which open while Na^+ is still entering. Eventually sufficient K^+ flows out for the membrane potential to revert to its original level. This process is complete within about 1 ms in a mammalian nerve, but a much longer time elapses before the original ionic distribution is restored by the membrane pump expelling Na^+ in exchange for K^+.

As sodium passes through an area of membrane (the 'active site'), it causes a flow of current to a hitherto inactive area just ahead of the impulse (local current action). The current flow causes this new area of membrane to depolarize partially, then it too becomes highly permeable to Na^+. The process continues and in this way an AP is propagated along the axonal length.

The larger the diameter of a nerve, the faster an AP passes along it. However, the greatest velocity (about 100 m s^{-1}) is attained in neurones which are invested with an insulating myelin sheath. In these fibres, Na^+ can gain entry only at areas where the axonal membrane is exposed, between gaps in the sheath (nodes of Ranvier). Now the local circuit current generated by the Na^+ entry acts far ahead of the active site and increases Na^+ entry at the next node – and so on. The active process therefore occurs in a series of jumps – 'saltatory conduction' – and the impulse travels faster than in the non-myelinated fibres (about 2 m s^{-1}), where the entire length of the axon will ultimately have undergone a change in Na^+ permeability. TFFFT

MCQ 32

In a single nerve fibre

1. subthreshold depolarizing stimuli cause a decrease in membrane excitability.
2. an absolute refractory period occurs for a few milliseconds after the passage of an action potential.
3. all propagated action potentials are normally constant in amplitude.
4. stimulated through electrodes placed on the axon, both orthodromic and antidromic impulses will be generated.
5. action potentials generated by excitatory neurotransmitters acting at the cell body will travel orthodromically only.

A nerve impulse can be generated by various stimuli; for example, by an excitatory neurotransmitter acting at the cell body, or by the passage of current through electrodes placed on the axon. In all cases a depolarization of the membrane is brought about at the point of stimulation (i.e. the negative potential is moved closer to zero). At threshold level (when the membrane potential reaches about $-55\,mV$) channels in the membrane open through which Na^+ flows very rapidly into the nerve. Transient subthreshold depolarizations do not open these channels but will briefly increase membrane excitability so that a second stimulus may summate with the first and thus initiate an action potential (AP).

An AP generated in an axon, unlike that originating at the cell body, is conducted in both directions away from the point of excitation. The impulse travels towards the terminal (orthodromically) and in the opposite direction (antidromically), in which case it will be extinguished when it reaches the cell body.

Within the period of the rising and falling phases of the AP (usually less than a millisecond) the affected area of membrane cannot be excited again, no matter how strong the stimulus (absolute refractory period). This is followed by the relative refractory period when K^+ is still flowing out and while the nerve membrane begins to regain its former excitability by pumping out the Na^+ which has gained access.

It is important to distinguish the all-or-none events occurring in a single nerve fibre, where all APs will have the same size, from those in a nerve trunk, where a compound AP can be measured by surface electrodes. These nerve trunks may contain many hundreds of nerve fibres with different conduction velocities, diameters and degrees of myelination. A just-threshold stimulus may excite only a fraction of the available fibres and the amplitude of the resulting compound AP will be smaller than when a stronger stimulus excites more fibres. The compound AP may thus be graded with respect to stimulus strength or drug effect and may show complex waveforms when fibres of different conduction velocity are stimulated. FFTTT

Local anaesthetic activity is possessed by

1. **propranolol.**
2. **gallamine.**
3. **mecamylamine.**
4. **chlorpromazine.**
5. **diphenhydramine.**

In order to produce local anaesthesia, drugs must penetrate the lipid barriers around axons. Most clinically used local anaesthetics are secondary or tertiary amines and, at physiological pH, both charged and non-charged forms of the molecule exist, the proportions depending on the pH of the environment and the pK_a (acid dissociation constant) of the molecule. The non-ionized (and hence lipid-soluble) form penetrates axonal membranes. A proportion of the intracellular drug ionizes and this cationic form may compete with Ca^{2+} which is involved in the opening of the Na^+ channel. The local anaesthetic thus prevents the transient increase in sodium permeability which is crucial in generating the rising phase of the action potential.

Various methods are used to assess local anaesthetic activity. They range from the direct application of a drug to electrically stimulated, desheathed nerve trunks to drug injection intradermally and the assessment of activity against mechanically induced pain (e.g. a pin prick). In these tests local anaesthesia can be obtained in varying degrees because many nerve fibres are involved; in some conduction will be blocked, while in others the action potential will propagate normally. Only rarely will tests involve single nerve fibres, in which case the local anaesthetic would completely abolish the action potential or leave it unaffected (since it is an all-or-none event).

Although four of the above drugs can be shown to be local anaesthetics, they are never used for this purpose because they have other major pharmacological actions:

(a) **Mecamylamine** blocks nicotinic receptors in ganglia.
(b) **Chlorpromazine** blocks many receptor types but owes its major tranquillizing activity to dopamine receptor blockade in the CNS.
(c) **Diphenhydramine** is a histamine H_1-receptor blocker.
(d) **Propranolol** is a β-adrenoceptor blocker having antianginal, anti-hypertensive and antidysrhythmic actions (though it could be argued that the last effect may involve some local anaesthesia of cardiac conducting tissue).

Gallamine, an antagonist of acetylcholine at the nicotinic receptors of the neuromuscular junction, is not a local anaesthetic, presumably because its three quaternary nitrogen groups confer such a low lipid solubility that it fails to penetrate the axonal membranes. TFTTT

MCQ 34

Local anaesthetics will produce

1. spinal anaesthesia if injected into the spinal cord.
2. spinal anaesthesia if hyperbaric solutions are injected into the cisterna magna.
3. epidural anaesthesia when injected intrathecally in the lower lumbar region.
4. anaesthesia restricted to the spinal segment at the level of injection when infiltrated between periosteal and dural layers.
5. no anaesthesia if introduced into the cerebrospinal fluid.

The brain and spinal cord are protected within their bony compartments by membranes (meninges). They are further cushioned by the cerebrospinal fluid (CSF), which fills the space between the closely investing pia and the looser arachnoid membranes. The more fibrous and tougher dura is the outer membrane. Cerebrospinal fluid is formed by the choroid plexuses (especially in the lateral ventricles) and fills both the ventricles and the intercommunicating subarachnoid space (between the pia and arachnoid). Dilatations of the subarachnoid space (cisternae) occur at intervals; of particular note is the cisterna magna between the medulla and the undersurface of the cerebellum.

Regional anaesthesia can be produced by introducing local anaesthetic solutions into the CSF. Injections must never be made into the spinal cord itself because of the damage which may be caused by the needle. To minimize this risk, injections are often made through the theca (sheath) into the lower lumbar region below the level at which the spinal cord terminates. Solutions less dense (hypobaric) than the CSF will rise and produce anaesthesia above the site of injection. By contrast, hyperbaric solutions will fall and produce spinal anaesthesia if injected into the cisterna magna (provided that the patient is not standing on his head!).

Since the dura is not in contact with the CSF, epidural anaesthesia will occur with injections made between the periosteal (the inside surface of the bony compartment) and dural layers. The drug will remain localized at the site of injection and thus affect only those nerves leaving the spinal cord at the level of injection. FTFTF

The addition of a pharmacologically effective concentration of **lignocaine** *to an isolated vas deferens preparation would reduce the response to*

1. transmural electrical stimulation.
2. hypogastric nerve stimulation.
3. **tyramine.**
4. **noradrenaline.**
5. **potassium chloride.**

The isolated vas deferens is frequently used to assess drug effects on noradrenergic neurotransmission. It can be dissected out with its accompanying hypogastric nerve, stimulation of which ultimately causes a release of noradrenaline (NA) from the postganglionic nerve terminals onto the smooth muscle. Unlike most sympathetic nerve supplies, ganglia occur in this pathway very close to the smooth muscle. Therefore the effects of hypogastric nerve stimulation can be greatly reduced by ganglion blocking drugs.

The vas deferens can be removed without its attached nerve trunk and will respond to shocks delivered through parallel platinum wires placed close to it in the organ bath. With short pulse widths (0.5 ms) so as not to excite muscle cells directly, the postganglionic nerves which remain embedded in the muscle are stimulated and release NA, which produces a contractile response from the muscle. These events are blocked by local anaesthetic drugs (e.g. **lignocaine**). **Tetrodotoxin**, a poison from the puffer fish, is one of the most active substances known in blocking neuronal sodium channels, thereby producing a 'local anaesthetic' effect. It is often used experimentally to demonstrate that events induced by electrical stimulation are mediated by neuronal actions and are not due to a direct effect on muscle fibres. **Tetrodotoxin** has an advantage over local anaesthetics for this purpose in that it has very few other effects at concentrations which block sodium channels.

Most local anaesthetics will not reduce responses to exogenous **NA**, which acts directly on the smooth muscle α-adrenoceptors to cause contraction. **Tyramine** causes a contraction by entering the nerve through the amine uptake mechanism and displacing endogenous NA, which then causes a contraction. It is worthwhile noting that **cocaine** (a local anaesthetic which, in addition, blocks the amine uptake mechanism in noradrenergic nerves) will potentiate exogenous **NA** by preventing its removal from the synapse by the uptake mechanism. **Tyramine** would be blocked by **cocaine** since its access to the endogenous NA stores is prevented.

A high concentration of potassium ions in the extracellular fluid will disturb the ionic balance across the muscle membrane, cause depolarization and hence contraction of the muscle. Local anaesthetics do not modify this action. TTFFF

MCQ 36

Local anaesthetic solutions frequently contain additives such as **adrenaline** *or* **felypressin,** *both of which*

1. will prolong the duration of local anaesthesia.
2. will increase the force of cardiac contraction if inadvertently given intravenously.
3. will be equally safe in patients taking monamine oxidase inhibitors.
4. may cause anaphylactic reactions.
5. are sympathomimetic amines.

Wherever local anaesthetics are injected, their action is usually terminated by absorption into blood vessels and removal from the site of injection by the blood flow. Thus any drug which constricts blood vessels will delay removal and prolong the local anaesthesia. Many local anaesthetics are themselves vasodilators. They are, therefore, given with the sympathomimetic amine **adrenaline** or with **felypressin** (a synthetic octapeptide), both of which cause vasoconstriction and so prolong local anaesthesia.

Vasoconstrictor additives are not without dangers. The pressor effects of **noradrenaline** may be greatly increased in patients taking tricyclic antidepressants like **imipramine** (which block the neuronal uptake of noradrenaline). Monoamine oxidase inhibitors (also used as antidepressants) might be expected to intensify the action of **adrenaline** or **noradrenaline** but in practice the effect is clinically insignificant. **Felypressin** interacts with neither type of antidepressant.

Adrenaline and **noradrenaline**, with their ability to stimulate both α- and β-adrenoceptors, constrict blood vessels (α) and stimulate the heart (β), while **felypressin** constricts blood vessels by another mechanism and has no effect on the heart.

Anaphylactic reactions occur when antigens (large molecular weight substances; typically protein) bind to complementary antibodies. This triggers the release of autacoids (such as histamine and arachidonic acid metabolites) with powerful actions on the cardiovascular and respiratory systems. **Adrenaline** is not antigenic (note that it occurs naturally and is released from the adrenal medulla). In fact, it is often used in the treatment of true anaphylactic emergencies because of its ability to dilate the bronchioles and stimulate the cardiovascular system. **Felypressin**, although a peptide, has a low molecular weight and is therefore unlikely to be antigenic. TFTFF

Applied locally to the cornea, cocaine *is likely to produce*

1. mydriasis.
2. cycloplegia.
3. widening of the palpebral fissure.
4. abolition of the corneal reflex.
5. paralysis of the external ocular muscles.

The local anaesthetic activity of **cocaine** causes inhibition of the corneal reflex since the sensory pathways will no longer conduct the stimulus from the touch receptors in the cornea and the blink reflex is therefore abolished. Anaesthesia is unlikely to extend to the iris as penetration through the aqueous humour of a sufficiently high concentration of **cocaine** is unusual. The extraocular muscles are innervated by myelinated somatic nerves, conduction in which will only be blocked by a higher concentration of local anaesthetic than would normally be used.

Mydriasis (pupillary dilatation) may be produced either by the relaxation of the inner circular muscles or by the contraction of the outer radial muscles of the iris. The circular muscles are normally partially contracted because their parasympathetic nerves are constantly active and release acetylcholine onto muscarinic receptors. Thus an atropinic drug will dilate the pupil by antagonizing acetylcholine. Radial muscle contraction occurs when its α-adrenoceptors are stimulated (e.g. by noradrenaline released from the sympathetic nerves).

Cocaine, at concentrations about 1000 times less than those needed to produce local anaesthesia, will inhibit the neuronal uptake process (uptake$_1$) which normally prevents an accumulation of noradrenaline in the synaptic cleft. **Cocaine** therefore enhances the effects of sympathetic nerve activity and causes mydriasis.

The palpebral fissure (distance between the upper and lower lids) is controlled both by cholinergic nerves to skeletal muscles and by noradrenergic nerves, the latter acting on a smooth muscle component of the upper lid. Potentiation of the effects of noradrenaline causes this muscle to contract and widens the palpebral fissure.

Cycloplegia (paralysis of accommodation) is not caused by **cocaine** since the shape of the lens is controlled by the ciliary muscles, which are cholinergically innervated. Since they are located behind the iris, local anaesthesia is even less likely to extend this far into the eye. TFTTF

MCQ 38

The local anaesthetic agent

1. **prilocaine** may be dangerous in a patient suffering from grossly impaired respiration.
2. **cinchocaine** will inhibit plasma cholinesterase.
3. **lignocaine** is also used in the treatment of epilepsy.
4. **cocaine** is restricted to uses involving surface anaesthesia.
5. **benzocaine** is superior to **lignocaine** for infiltration anaesthesia.

Clinically useful local anaesthetics nearly all contain an aromatic ring linked to an amino residue. The linkage may be through ester, amide, urea, ketone or ether groups. **Lignocaine** (also known as **lidocaine**, **Xylocaine** or **Xylotox**) is an amide, widely used for surface, infiltration, regional, epidural and spinal anaesthesia. It is also given by i.v. infusion for the treatment of certain cardiac dysrhythmias. **Lignocaine** is not normally used against epilepsy (indeed, overdose can produce convulsions), but it has been used occasionally to control the convulsions of status epilepticus, though **diazepam** would be preferred.

Cocaine has an ester link and penetrates mucous membranes better than most local anaesthetics. Its use is restricted to anaesthesia of the nose, throat and, occasionally, the cornea because of its potential cardiotoxicity and its liability to cause psychological dependence on repeated use. For most other applications, other local anaesthetics are as good and are not subject to the tight legislative restrictions applied in most countries.

Benzocaine also has an ester link, but is only slightly soluble in water and is applied in dusting powders or oily solutions to skin surfaces, where it produces sustained anaesthesia as a consequence of its slow absorption.

Prilocaine, which like **lignocaine** has an amide link, is metabolized to *o*-toluidine. *o*-Toluidine then converts haemoglobin to an oxidized form (methaemoglobin) which cannot carry oxygen. If tissue oxygenation is already marginal, for example through reduced respiratory function, a further reduction in oxygen delivery to the tissues would be very undesirable.

Cinchocaine (**dibucaine**), also an amide, is one of the most potent, most toxic and longest lasting local anaesthetics. Its activity as an inhibitor of plasma cholinesterase has been employed in tests on patients to discover if, through a genetic abnormality, their plasma cholinesterase is abnormal. Such patients metabolize the usually short-acting neuromuscular blocking agent **succinylcholine** very slowly and its paralysing action is therefore dangerously prolonged. TTFTF

Toxic hazards with local anaesthetics given by injection include

1. occasional allergic reactions causing sudden collapse.
2. stimulation of the CNS.
3. damage to veins because of the alkaline nature of the solutions.
4. spasm of the digital artery if injected into the finger.
5. physical dependence on repeated administration.

Allergic reactions such as dermatitis, asthma and even systemic anaphylaxis may occur in a few patients. Such reactions demand previous exposure to the drug because sensitization occurs through the formation of antibodies. This is especially likely to occur when the skin is exposed to the drug and so dental practitioners in particular must be cautious. Allergic reactions in patients may be avoided by using a different local anaesthetic, since allergy is often specific to a single chemical structure or group. For instance, a patient allergic to a local anaesthetic with an amide link may cross-react with other amides (**lignocaine**, **prilocaine**) but is less likely to react with, for example, **amethocaine**, which has an ester link.

Local anaesthetic solutions are not highly alkaline. It is solutions of barbiturates which may cause vascular damage because of their alkaline nature.

Vasoconstriction and arterial spasm are unlikely with local anaesthetics alone since (with the exception of **cocaine**) these cause dilatation of blood vessels or have little effect. The danger of spasm in arteries of the extremities arises from the **adrenaline** which may have been incorporated into the local anaesthetic solution. Therefore solutions of anaesthetic 'with vasoconstrictor' should not be injected into extremities.

No local anaesthetic given by injection has been reported to cause physical dependence. **Cocaine** is abused (by repeated surface application to the nasal mucosa, for example – 'cocaine sniffing') but does not produce physical dependence since no withdrawal syndrome occurs when **cocaine** use is stopped. Psychological dependence may occur, however. Of even greater abuse potential is **cocaine** in the form of its free base known as 'crack'.

All local anaesthetics will penetrate the blood–brain barrier into the CNS and will produce convulsions if given in sufficient quantity. TTFFF

Peripheral Cholinergic Nervous Systems

Neurotransmission at cholinergic nerve terminals will be impaired by

1. **hemicholinium** because it reduces choline uptake.
2. **botulinum toxin** because it rapidly depletes transmitter stores.
3. **black widow spider venom** because it blocks axonal sodium channels.
4. **styryl pyridines** because they inhibit choline acetylase.
5. **6-hydroxydopamine** because it causes neuronal destruction.

All cholinergic nerves possess a number of biological properties in common.

(a) An active axonal membrane transport system accumulates choline from the extracellular fluid. Dietary choline is usually available in adequate quantities, but choline can be synthesized in the liver by progressive methylation of serine using the *S*-adenosylmethionine methyl donor system.

(b) An enzymic process involving choline acetylase and acetyl-coenzyme A converts choline to acetylcholine (ACh).

(c) Intracellular vesicles take up and store ACh, thus protecting it from destruction (hydrolysis).

(d) A coupling mechanism is present whereby a depolarizing stimulus causes the vesicular and neuronal membranes to fuse and to liberate ACh and other vesicular contents into the synaptic cleft.

(e) A recycling process exists whereby vesicles are renewed after discharging their contents.

Hemicholinium inhibits choline uptake in a competitive manner and its effect can, therefore, be overcome by adding excess choline. **Triethylcholine** has a similar effect though it may, in addition, be converted to a false transmitter, acetyltriethylcholine.

Styryl pyridines inhibit choline acetylase.

Botulinum toxin binds strongly to the ganglioside components of the terminal membrane, prevents vesicles fusing with the neuronal membrane and hence prevents ACh release.

Black widow spider venom interrupts the vesicle recycling process and thus causes a failure to replace used vesicles, depletion of neuronal ACh and hence transmission failure.

6-Hydroxydopamine does not affect cholinergic nerves. The neuronal destruction which it causes is restricted to catecholaminergic nerves because they alone possess a neuronal uptake mechanism (uptake$_1$) able to concentrate **6-hydroxydopamine** within the nerve to the level required for neuronal damage to be produced.

None of these drugs has a clinical application but all have been used in studies of neurotransmission.

Botulinum toxin may be encountered in, for example, tinned meats (*Clostridium botulinum* is anaerobic) and leads to botulism, a rare condition with a high mortality rate. Treatment requires the use of antibodies to the toxin and may involve life-support systems because of respiratory failure since skeletal muscle is paralysed. Attempts may be made to protect people who work with **botulinum toxin**, either by giving antibodies or else a toxoid (to confer active immunity). The toxin is known to have been studied as an agent of biological warfare. TFFTF

MCQ 41

Receptors stimulated by acetylcholine

1. are designated muscarinic or nicotinic, depending on whether they are selectively stimulated by the alkaloids **muscarine** or **nicotine**.
2. may be located at sites where they are not normally exposed to released neurotransmitter.
3. which promote gastric acid secretion and intestinal muscle contraction are classified as muscarinic M_1-receptors.
4. are found on cholinergic nerve endings, where they modulate neurotransmitter release.
5. are found on sensory ganglion cells.

By definition, cholinergic nerves contain the neurotransmitter acetylcholine (ACh) and are found in peripheral and central nervous systems. In some neurones other substances, for example peptides, coexist with and seem to be released simultaneously with ACh; these substances may also play important roles in impulse transmission. The major peripheral cholinergic pathways are:

(a) in the efferent autonomic system (preganglionic sympathetic and parasympathetic; sympathetic nerves to the adrenal medulla; postganglionic parasympathetic fibres);
(b) in the somatic efferents to skeletal muscle.

Other cholinergic fibres run in the sympathetic supply to, for example, sweat glands (but most postganglionic sympathetic nerves are noradrenergic). By contrast, afferent (sensory) nerves use different transmitters, for example peptides, such as substance P. The cell bodies of sensory nerves lie in the dorsal root ganglia adjacent to the spinal cord but have no synaptic contacts with other nerves and therefore do not possess cholinoceptors.

Cholinoceptors are found on all cells innervated by cholinergic nerves and on some cells which are not, for example vascular endothelial cells. They are also present on terminals of cholinergic and other neurones. Stimulation of these presynaptic receptors affects the release of neurotransmitters (e.g. increasing the output of ACh from somatic nerves to skeletal muscle; decreasing the noradrenaline release from sympathetic postganglionic fibres).

Cholinoceptors are placed in two major classes according to whether they are stimulated by **nicotine** or **muscarine**. In the periphery, nicotinic receptors are found principally on cells in autonomic ganglia and the adrenal medulla (blocked by e.g. **hexamethonium**) and on skeletal muscle end-plates (blocked by e.g. **gallamine**). At other locations cholinoceptors are muscarinic, subdivided into M_1 and M_2 according to the selectivity of ligands. M_1-receptors are present in sympathetic ganglia and on gastric cells secreting HCl, are stimulated by **McN-A-343** (4-(*m*-chlorophenyl-carbamoyloxy)-2-butyntrimethylammonium chloride) and blocked by **pirenzipine**. M_2-receptors represent most of the remaining muscarinic receptors, for which no highly selective ligands are yet known. It should

continued on next page

be noted that other subtypes have been proposed on the basis of differences in the binding characteristics of drugs either to membrane fragments or to isolated tissue proteins, though their functional roles remain in doubt.

Cholinoceptor agonists include choline esters (e.g. **carbachol**), naturally occurring alkaloids from plants (**pilocarpine**) and synthetic chemicals (**furmethide**). Drugs which inhibit the hydrolysis of ACh (anticholinesterases) may also exhibit cholinomimetic effects. TTFTF

MCQ 42

Choline esters used therapeutically include

1. **bethanechol**, given by mouth in cases of postoperative abdominal distension.
2. **methacholine**, given subcutaneously to cause bradycardia.
3. **carbachol**, given intravenously to relieve paralytic ileus.
4. **bethanechol**, given subcutaneously to combat acute urinary retention.
5. **carbachol**, given orally to patients with myasthenia gravis.

All cholinomimetic agents will mimic, in certain respects, the actions of acetylcholine (ACh), but degrees of selectivity on muscarinic or nicotinic receptors are apparent. **Carbachol, methacholine** and **bethanechol** are all adequate agonists at muscarinic receptors and may be used clinically because of this property. At higher doses **carbachol** also has a stimulant action on nicotinic receptors and may cause sympathetic ganglion excitation and skeletal muscle contraction. However, **carbachol** is still employed clinically because of its resistance to hydrolysis. **Carbachol** may be used for ophthalmic purposes, when it is instilled into the conjunctival sac (often with a wetting agent to improve penetration) in the treatment of non-congestive wide-angle glaucoma.

Methacholine, with little nicotinic activity, has a relatively pronounced effect on the muscarinic receptors of the cardiovascular system and causes a fall in blood pressure with a compensatory tachycardia. Thus, although its direct action on the sinoatrial node would lead to bradycardia, the reflex response to the fall in blood pressure overrides this effect.

Bethanechol is also resistant to hydrolysis by cholinesterase and is active when taken by mouth, in spite of being, like all choline esters, a quaternary nitrogen compound. It is devoid of nicotinic activity, has less marked effects on the cardiovascular system than **methacholine** and is used in the treatment of gut or bladder atony. An alternative treatment would be to use an anticholinesterase agent such as **neostigmine**, which preserves from destruction the ACh released from the parasympathetic fibres which innervate the gut and bladder.

Muscarinic cholinoceptors have been subdivided into two major functional groups, designated M_1 and M_2. Several drugs are known which possess a higher affinity for M_1-receptors but, as yet, no selective ligands for M_2-receptors have been discovered. None of the choline esters mentioned above is selective between muscarinic receptors. These drugs differ in potency on M_2-receptors, in susceptibility to hydrolysis and in relative activity on nicotinic receptors. Nonetheless, the search for selective agonists and antagonists continues, with impetus from the findings that some antagonists can discriminate between M_2-muscarinic receptors in gut, atria and lung even though their selectivity is low, suggesting that this group of receptors is not homogeneous. TFFTF

Pilocarpine *will produce*

1. sweating.
2. lachrymation.
3. emesis.
4. increased intraocular pressure.
5. dry mouth.

Pilocarpine is a natural alkaloid from the leaves of a South American shrub and is an agonist at muscarinic cholinoceptors, as are the alkaloids **muscarine** (from a poisonous species of mushroom) and **arecoline** (from betel nuts). All these substances will, in various degrees, mimic the effects of acetylcholine released from autonomic postganglionic cholinergic nerves and may be termed parasympathomimetic. **Pilocarpine** stimulates the sweat glands, innervated by cholinergic sympathetic nerves. It is a powerful diaphoretic drug which, after s.c. injection, may cause the secretion of up to 2 litres of sweat. It also causes lachrymation. The tear secretions in rats contain a red pigment and the drug, therefore, produces chromodacryorrhesis ('bloody tears'). It increases salivary secretion (muscarinic stimulation) and if given by mouth may cause emesis (vomiting).

    Pilocarpine has complex effects on the cardiovascular system and usually causes a small vasodepressor response after i.v. injection. However, after nicotinic ganglion blockade, it produces a rise in blood pressure which is attenuated by **atropine**. It is therefore possible that, in addition to its parasympathomimetic actions on M_2-receptors, **pilocarpine** stimulates muscarinic M_1-receptors in sympathetic ganglia and this produces a sympathomimetic response like the preferential M_1-receptor agonist **McN-A-343** (4-(m-chlorophenylcarbamoyloxy)-2-butyntrimethylammonium chloride). This suggestion is supported by the observation that α-adrenoceptor blocking drugs, which inhibit the vasoconstrictor action of **noradrenaline** block the rise in blood pressure to **pilocarpine**.

    Pilocarpine finds a use in the treatment of glaucoma, where it constricts the pupil (miosis), improving drainage of the aqueous humour through the canal of Schlemm and thereby reducing intraocular pressure. It is used as an eye-drop or as a sustained release preparation (a lamella: a small plastic disc impregnated with **pilocarpine**, placed under the lower eyelid and renewed weekly). Unlike choline esters (**acetylcholine**, **methacholine** and **carbachol**), which are quaternary nitrogen compounds, poorly lipid-soluble and therefore unable to penetrate the cornea very well, **pilocarpine** is a tertiary amine, exists in ionized and non-ionized forms ($pK_a = 6.9$) and will therefore penetrate readily.

    Neither **arecoline** nor **muscarine** is used clinically. It should be noted that poisoning caused by species of mushroom which contain **muscarine** may be due to the presence of other toxic substances. Thus treatment with **atropine** will effectively counter the salivation, lachrymation, bronchospasm etc. due to **muscarine**. However, *Amanita muscaria* contains isoxazoles which cause hallucinations and which themselves have antagonistic effects against acetylcholine. Other species contain amatoxins (cyclic octapeptides) which block messenger RNA synthesis and cause cell death. **Atropine** is not an antidote to such poisons. TTTFF

MCQ 44

Cholinoceptors in sympathetic ganglia may be

1. blocked by **hexamethonium**.
2. blocked by **atropine**.
3. blocked by **McN-A-343**.
4. stimulated by **carbachol**.
5. stimulated by **dopamine**.

Sympathetic ganglionic transmission is known to involve a more complex set of events than mere liberation of acetylcholine (ACh) from preganglionic terminals onto nicotinic receptors on the cell bodies. For instance, biochemical analyses reveal the presence of a variety of peptides (substance P, angiotensin) in nerve terminals which may be released by neuronal activity and may affect the transmission process. There are also monoamine-containing cells (probably dopaminergic) within ganglia which appear to exert inhibitory effects on transmission. Electrophysiological measurements on cell bodies reveal that preganglionic stimulation causes complex changes involving at least three separate neurotransmitters; and receptor analyses show that binding sites exist for ACh, monoamines and several peptides, all of which may play important roles in ganglionic transmission.

Physiologically important nicotinic cholinoceptors in ganglia are mainly responsible for the excitatory postsynaptic potential and hence the propagated action potential in postganglionic fibres. These receptors are different from their counterparts in skeletal muscle, especially in their affinity for antagonists (e.g. **hexamethonium** selectively affects ganglia). Some antagonists are thought to compete with ACh for the receptor site (**mecamylamine, trimetaphan**) but others are known to block the receptor-associated ion channel (**hexamethonium, pempidine**). Channel blockade accounts for the increasing effectiveness of these drugs when the agonist concentration is raised, because more open channels then become available (use-dependent block).

Muscarinic receptors with excitatory functions have also been found on ganglion cells though their physiological role is unclear. These receptors can be stimulated by **carbachol** and blocked by **atropine**. They appear to belong to the M_1-subclass since they are also stimulated by the experimental drug **McN-A-343** (4-(*m*-chlorophenylcarbamoyloxy)-2-butyntrimethylammonium chloride), which is virtually devoid of activity at M_2-muscarinic sites. Thus its i.v. injection causes tachycardia and a rise in blood pressure due to stimulation of sympathetic ganglia which culminates in release of noradrenaline at the heart and blood vessels. This ganglion stimulant action is blocked by **atropine** but unaffected by **hexamethonium**. The virtual absence of M_1-muscarinic receptors in parasympathetic ganglia (and in most of the innervated organs) means that **McN-A-343** has little parasympathomimetic activity.

Studies of electrical changes induced by endogenous or exogenous amines and peptides present a confusing picture which illustrates the complexities of ganglionic transmission. In some ganglia **substance P** has excitatory actions and may facilitate transmission by presynaptic effects. By contrast, **enkephalins** are inhibitory, as is **dopamine**. All these substances act on their own receptor types. The changes brought about by peptides and amines are modulatory, rather than primary, and it should be realized that drugs which block nicotinic receptors can totally inhibit ganglionic transmission. TTFTF

The logical consequences of administering a ganglion blocking drug to man include

1. postural hypotension.
2. diarrhoea.
3. paralysis of accommodation.
4. increased salivation.
5. skeletal muscle weakness.

Ganglion blocking drugs (e.g. **hexamethonium, pempidine, mecamylamine**) reduce all autonomic activity by inhibiting the nicotinic actions of acetylcholine in sympathetic and parasympathetic ganglia. Since vascular innervation and the maintenance of peripheral resistance are mediated almost entirely through sympathetic vasoconstrictor nerves, a fall in systemic arterial pressure is inevitable when these pathways are interrupted. Normally, in a person changing from a recumbent to an upright posture, the reduction in venous return (and consequent fall in cardiac output and blood pressure) is rapidly compensated by reflex activity. The reflexes cause an increased efferent sympathetic discharge, raising total peripheral resistance. Ganglion blocking drugs will reduce this reflex activity and 'postural hypotension' results. Many other drugs which interfere with the integrity of the sympathetic nervous system also reduce reflex activity, though possibly to a lesser extent.

In the intestine both the contractile (parasympathetic) and the relaxant (sympathetic) components of neuronal control will be reduced by ganglion blockade. However, constipation occurs because of removal of the normally dominant parasympathetic control which stimulates propulsive movements.

In the eye, accommodation is controlled by the parasympathetic supply to the ciliary muscles. These muscles will be relaxed during ganglion blockade, producing a lens fixed for distant vision.

Salivary secretions are induced by both sympathetic and parasympathetic stimulation and will be reduced after ganglion blockade. The parasympathetic is the more important – hence the severe dry mouth after drugs with atropine-like actions (e.g. **atropine** itself or tricyclic antidepressants like **desmethylimipramine**).

Skeletal muscles are innervated by motor nerves which do not have ganglia. Furthermore, the nicotinic receptors at the neuromuscular junction are of a different type from those at the ganglia; voluntary muscle will thus be unaffected by most ganglion blocking drugs although, in large doses, **mecamylamine** may produce neuromuscular blockade. **Mecamylamine** has a long duration of action because it is largely unmetabolized and excreted slowly by the kidney. Being a secondary amine, it is absorbed well from the gut and also passes readily into the CNS, where it can act to cause tremor, mental confusion, seizures etc. Nowadays ganglion blocking drugs are rarely used clinically, although the short-acting sulphonium compound **trimetaphan** is occasionally used to treat hypertensive crises or to create a 'bloodless' field during surgery by lowering the blood pressure. TFTFF

In experiments using neuromuscular blocking agents

1. **decamethonium** and **tubocurarine** both cause relaxation of frog rectus abdominis muscle.
2. **pancuronium** inhibits the effects of both sciatic nerve stimulation and intra-arterial **acetylcholine** on cat tibialis muscle.
3. the mechanism of action of **decamethonium** and **gallamine** is identical on rat phrenic nerve–diaphragm preparation.
4. **atropine** prevents the spastic paralysis induced by **succinylcholine** in the chick.
5. tetanic contractions of cat tibialis muscle cannot be sustained when either **tubocurarine** or **succinylcholine** is given.

Drugs could prevent neuromuscular transmission by presynaptic or postsynaptic actions. By common usage the term neuromuscular blockade refers to drugs which act mainly postsynaptically to cause failure of skeletal muscle to respond to somatic nerve stimulation. Many drugs with this action are used clinically as muscle relaxants during surgery. They share the property of binding to nicotinic receptor sites but differ in potency, in selectivity (e.g. **tubocurarine** also binds to ganglionic nicotinic receptors) and in their mode of action (e.g. **pancuronium** is a competitive antagonist; **succinylcholine**, a partial agonist). Skeletal muscle from different locations and from different species has been used to investigate these drugs; experiments have been done *in vivo* and *in vitro* and measured parameters include: muscle contraction; electrical activity at synapses; and opening and closing of ion channels at motor end-plates.

The simplest experiments are performed on frog isolated muscle, such as strips of the rectus abdominis muscle, which overlies the abdomen. Unlike mammalian muscle, this contracts slowly when nicotinic receptors are stimulated and the contraction is well maintained. Therefore full agonists (e.g. **acetylcholine**; **ACh**) and partial agonists (e.g. **decamethonium**) cause contracture, a response inhibited by competitive antagonists like **tubocurarine**. Avian muscle similarly exhibits sustained contracture with agonists; **succinylcholine** causes spastic paralysis when injected into the chick, an effect which can be countered by nicotinic blockers but not by **atropine**, a muscarinic antagonist.

The diaphragm is a skeletal muscle which responds with a brief contracture (twitch) to intermittent stimulation of the phrenic nerve. The effect of neuromuscular blockers is gradually to diminish the amplitude of evoked twitches. **Gallamine** competes with released ACh for nicotinic receptors, thereby diminishing the twitch. The partial agonist **succinylcholine**, however, is a depolarizing agent which first stimulates the receptors, potentiating the twitch during its initial stages, but later reducing the twitch amplitude when the persisting end-plate depolarization causes refractoriness to released ACh.

The measurement of tibialis muscle contractions to sciatic nerve stimulation, or to intra-arterial **ACh**, in the cat permits drugs to be assessed *in vivo*. Twitches caused by low-frequency stimulation (0.1 Hz), as well as the

continued on next page

contractions to injected **ACh**, are inhibited by competitive nicotinic blockers (e.g. **pancuronium**). Tetanic contractions evoked by high frequencies (e.g. 30 Hz) can be used to distinguish between competitive and depolarizing agents, the former causing contractions to fade during the period of stimulation, the latter permitting tension to be maintained. One possible explanation for the fade is that presynaptic nicotinic receptors are involved in a positive feedback role: their stimulation by released ACh permits larger amounts of neurotransmitter to be released but, if they are blocked, transmitter output falls; hence the muscle receives insufficient ACh to maintain its tension. FTFFF

Succinylcholine *and* tubocurarine

1. will cause flaccid paralysis and spastic paralysis respectively in the chick.
2. will not produce skeletal muscle relaxation if given orally.
3. are not metabolized by acetylcholinesterase.
4. will both cause flaccid paralysis of skeletal muscle in cat and man.
5. act exclusively on skeletal muscle nicotinic receptors.

These drugs owe their clinical use as muscle relaxants in surgery to their interaction with nicotinic receptors in skeletal muscle. However, **tubocurarine** antagonizes the effects of acetylcholine (ACh) not only at these receptors but also at ganglionic nicotinic sites. It has been used, as a ganglion blocking drug, in animals in which the cerebral hemispheres have been destroyed, but, because of its ability to produce paralysis, written permission of the Home Secretary is required if **tubocurarine** or similar drugs are to be administered to conscious or anaesthetized animals in the UK.

The mode of action of these two drugs as muscle relaxants is different in man though the end effect (paralysis) is similar. **Succinylcholine** is a partial agonist and, particularly in avian and amphibian muscles which are not focally innervated, the pronounced agonist action leads to contracture and spastic paralysis (e.g. in the chick). The result of partial agonist activity in human and feline muscles is the brief fasciculations which often precede the flaccid paralysis. **Tubocurarine** produces flaccid paralysis in all species by competitive antagonism of ACh.

Both drugs possess positively charged (quaternary) nitrogen atoms (N^+), which confer poor lipid solubility and a general inability to pass through cell membranes (other than those in the glomerulus, which have large aqueous pores). Thus their absorption from the gastrointestinal tract is poor, as also is the ability of these drugs to gain access to the CNS from the bloodstream, although central nicotinic receptors can be affected if the blood–brain barrier is bypassed, for example by intracerebroventricular administration. **Succinylcholine** has a very short duration of action because, unlike **tubocurarine**, it is an ester and is rapidly hydrolysed by butyryl cholinesterase, an enzyme found principally in plasma. It should be noted that unusual sensitivity to **succinylcholine** is exhibited by some patients, in whom paralysis of respiratory muscles may occur for up to 1 h after administration of a dose the effects of which would normally be expected to last for less than 5 min. This is due to genetic abnormality, resulting in the possession of a deviant form of cholinesterase which fails to hydrolyse the drug. Compared with **succinylcholine**, most competitive blocking drugs have relatively long durations of action because little metabolism occurs and renal excretion accounts for their offset. However, **fazadinium** is almost totally metabolized in the liver and **atracurium** is degraded in the plasma, being chemically unstable at physiological pH. These factors account for their shorter duration of action and their less hazardous use in patients with compromised renal function. FTTTF

'Competitive' neuromuscular blocking drugs are used clinically to

1. relax visceral smooth muscle.
2. counteract the effects of **edrophonium** in myasthenic patients.
3. prevent abdominal skeletal muscle movements.
4. inhibit eyeball movements.
5. produce pupillary dilatation.

Neuromuscular blockers affect skeletal muscles and are used principally in surgery to cause relaxation, which enables muscles to be dissected more readily. Since high concentrations of general anaesthetics alone would be needed to produce the same gross effect, the use of a neuromuscular blocker enables a light anaesthesia to be maintained (and thus a low concentration of anaesthetic administered) while achieving muscular relaxation.

Neuromuscular blockers are not used to influence autonomic function (which controls, e.g. visceral tone and pupil size) though some, like **tubocurarine**, may additionally cause ganglion blockade.

Edrophonium is an anticholinesterase drug which combines with the anionic site on the enzyme and has a very short duration of action. Since myasthenia gravis involves an autoimmune destruction of nicotinic cholinoceptors on skeletal muscle, the prime symptoms involve skeletal muscle weakness. This is transiently relieved by **edrophonium**, which preserves acetylcholine from destruction and thus permits more nicotinic receptors to be activated. This is the basis of a diagnostic test and, since the drug's action is so short, no antidote is necessary. Longer-acting anticholinesterase agents (e.g. **neostigmine**) would be used for treatment of myasthenia gravis.

Note that longer-acting anticholinesterase drugs such as **neostigmine** may be used to reverse the neuromuscular blockade at the end of a surgical operation unless the final stitching procedure takes so long that the blockade is reversed by biotransformation or excretion of the neuromuscular blocker. With some neuromuscular blocking agents which have a relatively long duration of action (e.g. **pancuronium**), it is important to ensure that the anticholinesterase drug has a sufficiently long duration of action or its effects may wear off and neuromuscular blockade may return (paralysis of respiration) while the patient is back on the ward.

Although protracted effects of competitive blocking agents could be reversed by anticholinesterases, there was a clear advantage to be gained from the development of shorter-acting drugs. In some cases the promise of such drugs discovered in experiments using cats was not fulfilled when tested in man. However, **fazadinium** proved to have a short duration in clinical use, due to a rapid and almost total hepatic reduction of a diazolinkage in its structure. Even shorter in action is **atracurium**, a bisquaternary compound which, though stable in storage at acid pH, breaks down to inactive products by a Hoffmann degradation reaction at physiological pH. Thus both these drugs have advantages in patients with renal dysfunction who are undergoing surgery. FFTTF

MCQ 49

All anticholinesterase drugs may produce

1. stimulation followed by paralysis in ganglia.
2. parasympathomimetic effects.
3. direct or indirect effects on cholinoceptors in the CNS.
4. skeletal muscle paralysis.
5. increased sweating.

Three groups of anticholinesterase agent exist based on their interaction with the anionic and esteratic sites on the enzyme: (a) short-acting, easily reversible agents (e.g. **edrophonium**), which attach to the anionic site only; (b) longer-acting but still reversible agents (e.g. **neostigmine, physostigmine**), which attach to both sites and may also act as substrates for the enzyme; (c) 'irreversible' agents (e.g. the organophosphorus compounds such as **di-isopropyl fluorophosphonate** and **sarin**), which ultimately bind covalently to the esteratic site.

Many compounds in groups (a) and (b) are quaternary nitrogen compounds; they are therefore poorly lipid-soluble and fail to penetrate the blood–brain barrier. Hence the CNS is little affected by them. Compounds in the organophosphorus group (c) readily penetrate the CNS (and even penetrate unbroken skin).

All these compounds inhibit the enzymic hydrolysis of acetylcholine (ACh) and thus increase its concentration and activity at cholinoceptors. The peripheral effects of high concentrations of ACh will, therefore, be common to all the groups (e.g. parasympathomimetic actions: increased salivary, lachrymal and bronchial secretions; defaecation; increased intestinal activity). Although eccrine sweat glands are innervated by fibres which are anatomically sympathetic, these are, atypically, cholinergic and the glands have muscarinic receptors. Furthermore, ACh, at high concentrations, may produce depolarization blockade both at ganglia and at skeletal muscles. Therefore transmission may be inhibited at both these sites and skeletal muscle paralysis may eventually occur.

Muscarinic blockers and both ganglion and, possibly, neuromuscular blockers are used in the treatment of anticholinesterase poisoning. With the organophosphorus 'nerve gases' (**sarin, VX, tabun**), CNS depressants are also used. Furthermore, provided that treatment can be instituted within an hour of poisoning, drugs like **pralidoxime** should be given because they can prevent covalent binding of the organophosphorus compound to the esteratic site of the enzyme. TTFTT

Physostigmine *may be used to treat*

1. paralytic ileus.
2. parkinsonism.
3. atrial tachycardia.
4. gastric ulceration.
5. belladonna alkaloid poisoning.

The alkaloid **physostigmine** occurs naturally in the Calabar (ordeal) bean from West Africa. It is a competitive inhibitor of cholinesterase, being very slowly hydrolysed itself by the enzyme. Unlike its synthetic analogues **neostigmine** and **pyridostigmine**, **physostigmine** does not contain a positively charged (quaternary) nitrogen atom (N^+). Since its lipid solubility is, therefore, higher, the drug will be relatively well absorbed from the gut and will also gain access to the CNS.

Because acetylcholine (ACh) is preserved from hydrolysis in its presence, **physostigmine** is used to treat belladonna poisoning since the atropinic alkaloids in the plant are competitive antagonists of ACh at muscarinic receptors.

Both paralytic ileus and atrial tachycardia can be relieved by drugs which stimulate the muscarinic receptors of the gut and sinoatrial node respectively. Since it prevents destruction of ACh, **physostigmine** can be used though other anticholinesterase agents are often preferred.

Gastric ulceration will be made worse by measures which increase the secretion of HCl into the stomach, for example vagal stimulation or cholinomimetic drugs. Parkinson's disease, a condition of akinesia, tremor and rigidity, is associated with a destructive lesion of dopaminergic nerves in the nigrostriatal pathway with a resulting overactivity of functionally opposing cholinergic nerves acting through muscarinic receptors. Thus, in each case, **physostigmine** and other cholinomimetic drugs will worsen the condition. However, **physostigmine** has been used, though with little success, in the early stages of Alzheimer's disease in an attempt to improve memory. This condition, a type of senile dementia, has been associated with a reduction in cholinergic neurones, which explains why an anticholinesterase drug might be effective if it could restore cholinergic function. It should be noted, however, that other neurotransmitter systems can be affected in this disease.

The quaternary analogues, **pyridostigmine** and **neostigmine**, not only inhibit cholinesterases but have weak agonist activity at nicotinic sites. Therefore they are used for their effects on skeletal muscle such as in the treatment of myasthenia gravis or else in surgery to reverse the effects of competitive neuromuscular blocking agents. TFTFT

MCQ 51

Signs and symptoms of belladonna *poisoning include*

1. dry mouth and blurred vision.
2. tachycardia.
3. hot dry skin.
4. skin rash.
5. mydriasis.

The deadly nightshade plant (*Atropa belladonna*) has glossy black berries which are very attractive to children. They contain **atropine** and are a common cause of **atropine** poisoning. Henbane (*Hyoscyamus niger*) contains an alkaloid, **scopolamine** (**hyoscine**), which acts similarly to **atropine** in the periphery, although its effects on the CNS are different. Even when **atropine** has been used for ophthalmic purposes, poisoning has occurred due to systemic absorption of the drug after passage through the nasolachrymal duct. **Atropine** has a wide safety margin and antidotes to its effects are available so intoxication can be readily counteracted.

Most of the toxic effects can be predicted from a knowledge of the distribution and function of muscarinic cholinoceptors at which **atropine** is a competitive blocker. It can, therefore, be termed a 'parasympatholytic' agent. Salivation is inhibited so the patient has a dry burning mouth. This makes talking and swallowing difficult and the patient is thirsty. Vision is blurred as the ciliary muscles cannot contract to focus for near vision. Mydriasis (pupillary dilatation) and photophobia (sensitivity to light) are prominent since the circular muscle of the iris now fails to respond to its cholinergic innervation and the pupil dilates. In children especially, where the vagal tone is high, the heart rate increases (block of vagal tone) and the blood pressure may therefore rise. Hyperthermia occurs and the skin becomes hot and dry because the sympathetic cholinergic sweating mechanism is inhibited. A characteristic pink rash is seen, particularly on the face, neck and upper thorax, and patients are usually restless, excited and confused. **Scopolamine** produces CNS excitation too, but only when given in high doses or in patients suffering severe pain. When used in preanaesthetic medication, lower doses cause drowsiness, amnesia and fatigue.

The rational therapy for poisoning with either **atropine** or **scopolamine** is an anticholinesterase, which by preserving acetylcholine will permit the neurotransmitter to compete more effectively for the muscarinic receptors. **Physostigmine** is the preferred antidote since it can cross the blood–brain barrier and help alleviate the CNS effects of the toxic alkaloids. TTTTT

Atropine sulphate

1. causes mydriasis which may last for several days.
2. prevents the acetylcholine-induced release of catecholamines from the adrenal medulla.
3. inhibits the spastic paralysis caused by acetylcholine in the chick.
4. like **atropine methyl nitrate**, blocks muscarinic receptors in the CNS.
5. prevents the rise in blood pressure caused by muscarinic receptor stimulants acting on sympathetic ganglia.

Atropine is a competitive antagonist of acetylcholine (ACh) at all muscarinic receptors. **Atropine sulphate** is a simple salt (two atropine molecules are combined with each sulphate group) and as such will ionize in the body. The nature of the salt-forming acid is irrelevant except with regard to the molecular weight of the salt. However, **atropine methyl nitrate** is not a simple salt because the methyl group is bonded to the tertiary amino group of atropine, converting it to a quaternary nitrogen compound. Therefore **atropine methyl nitrate** is a polar compound which has a very restricted ability to penetrate cell membranes. In particular, it cannot cross the blood–brain barrier; thus CNS effects are not produced.

Since the circular muscle of the iris is parasympathetically innervated and is usually in a state of partial contraction, **atropine** antagonizes ACh, resulting in pupillary dilatation (mydriasis) which lasts for up to 7 days if **atropine** is instilled into the conjunctival sac. Other shorter-acting atropinic agents are available for ophthalmic use (e.g. **cyclopentolate**).

The cholinoceptors on the adrenal medulla and on chick skeletal muscle are nicotinic (though not identical with each other). Therefore **atropine** is ineffective at these sites.

Evidence has accumulated that different types of muscarinic receptor exist, the major groups being designated M_1 and M_2. Whilst no drugs are yet known with a high selectivity for M_2-receptors (which are more widely distributed), the M_1 type are preferentially stimulated by an experimental compound **McN-A-343** (4-(m-chlorophenylcarbamoyloxy)-2-butyntrimethyl-ammonium chloride) and blocked by **pirenzipine**. M_1-receptors occur in sympathetic ganglia, where stimulation leads to a sympathomimetic effect, and on oxyntic cells of the gastric mucosa, which secrete HCl. The injection of **McN-A-343** causes an increase in blood pressure and heart rate which is unaffected by nicotinic ganglion blockers but is prevented by atropinic agents. The physiological role of these ganglionic receptors is unclear; there is no evidence for their presence in the parasympathetic system, so **McN-A-343** is generally devoid of parasympathomimetic activity.

Atropine occurs naturally in *Atropa belladonna* (deadly nightshade). The consumption of this poisonous plant by rabbits has led over the years to the natural selection of a strain of rabbits with a plasma enzyme that destroys **atropine** (by hydrolysis) very rapidly. TFFFT

MCQ 53

Atropine-like activity in a drug

1. may be assessed using the frog rectus abdominis muscle.
2. means that the drug will selectively block muscarinic cholinoceptors.
3. may lead to its use in the treatment of parkinsonism.
4. may contraindicate its use in asthmatic patients.
5. may be counteracted by the administration of **scopolamine**.

Atropine-like activity means the drug will be a competitive antagonist of acetylcholine (ACh) at muscarinic receptors. However, possession of this property should not be taken to mean that the drug lacks other pharmacological actions (some of which could be apparent at concentrations lower than those required to block muscarinic receptors).

Parkinson's disease is thought to stem from a degeneration of the dopaminergic neurones in the nigrostriatal pathway, resulting in a relative overactivity of a cholinergic mechanism mediated through muscarinic receptors which is responsible for the disordered movement (tremor, rigidity). Atropinic agents (e.g. **ethopropazine**) thus reduce the cholinergic dominance and are beneficial.

Asthmatic patients, regardless of whether their asthma is provoked by allergens or other stimuli, often show increased sensitivity to many bronchoconstrictor agents (of which ACh is one). Furthermore, there is evidence of reflex parasympathetic activity in response to many stimuli. Since ACh will constrict bronchioles through muscarinic receptors, atropinic agents would help rather than harm an asthmatic patient.

The frog rectus abdominis muscle is mainly skeletal muscle (but is not focally innervated) and muscarinic receptors are involved to a very minor extent only. It would be inappropriate to test for atropinic activity using this muscle.

Scopolamine is chemically related to **atropine**; it too is parasympatholytic but has greater CNS depressant properties. **Atropine** is (±)-**hyoscyamine** and **scopolamine** is (−)-**hyoscine**. These alkaloids are found naturally in solanaceous plants (e.g. deadly nightshade, henbane) and are a cause of poisoning, especially in children.

The discovery of drugs with selectivity for muscarinic receptors in certain organs has led to a subdivision into M_1 and M_2 types. The M_2-receptors are more abundant and mediate most parasympathomimetic responses; they may not be a homogeneous group and further subdivision seems likely, though presently no highly selective drugs for these subtypes have been found. **Pirenzipine** is a selective antagonist for M_1-receptors and is being assessed for clinical use as an antiulcer agent since it can reduce the M_1-mediated release of HCl from oxyntic glands. The search for alternative atropine-like drugs therefore requires a variety of animal models, representing the different types of receptor which might be selectively blocked. FFTFF

Glaucoma

1. may be relieved by anticholinesterase drugs, which reduce the rate of formation of aqueous humour.
2. involves increased intraocular pressure and may lead to blindness.
3. of the narrow-angle type may be improved by miotics.
4. of the congenital type may require surgery.
5. may be precipitated in an acute form by mydriatic drugs.

Glaucoma is a painful condition caused by a rise in intraocular pressure due to accumulation of aqueous humour. If sufficiently high and prolonged, the pressure may damage the optic disc, leading to blindness. Some types of glaucoma (e.g. congenital) are best relieved by surgery; others, by drugs. Primary glaucoma is subdivided into narrow-angle and open-angle, according to the shape of the anterior chamber where reabsorption of the intraocular fluid occurs. Drugs may reduce the increased pressure either by decreasing the rate of production of aqueous humour from the epithelial cells of the ciliary body or by increasing its removal through the canal of Schlemm (a duct at the conjunction of the iris and cornea whose diameter is influenced by iris thickness). The patency of the trabecular network, a system of pores leading to and surrounding the canal, may be improved by changes in tone of the iris and ciliary muscles.

Drugs which cause miosis (pupillary constriction) are used to treat glaucoma. In miosis the iris muscle becomes thinner at its junction with the cornea and so increases the access of fluid to the trabecular network. Anticholinesterases (e.g. **physostigmine**) act by preserving acetylcholine (ACh) and thus potentiate its normal action to contract the circular muscle of the iris. For greater effectiveness, **physostigmine** may be used in combination with **pilocarpine** (a plant alkaloid which is a muscarinic cholinoceptor agonist). **Pilocarpine** is available as eye-drops or in a slow-release form – a lamella impregnated with the drug which is placed below the lower eyelid and renewed weekly. An effect on accommodation is likely to occur, especially with anticholinesterases, since the accumulation of ACh will cause contraction of the ciliary muscle, thereby fixing the focus of the lens for near vision.

Narrow-angle, sometimes called acute congestive, glaucoma often presents as an emergency. It will usually be treated with miotic drugs, though **acetazolamide** (a carbonic anhydrase inhibitor which reduces production of humour) or **mannitol** (an osmotic diuretic which causes intraocular dehydration) may be needed. In long-term management, surgery may be necessary, especially if adhesions develop between the iris and ciliary body.

Open-angle glaucoma too is responsive to miotics, but alternative drugs are often used in this condition. The long-acting β_1-adrenoceptor blocking agent **timolol** reduces the secretion of aqueous humour as, paradoxically, does **adrenaline**, which may additionally lower intraocular tissue volume by constricting blood vessels. However, **adrenaline** also produces mydriasis (by stimulating α-adrenoceptors on the radial muscle of the iris) which, unless countered with a miotic drug, could be dangerous since a thickened iris muscle may further restrict the outflow of aqueous humour. FTTTT

MCQ 55

Pupillary dilatation and diminished pupillary light reflex would be the likely consequence of instilling into the conjunctival sac a solution of

1. lignocaine.
2. cocaine.
3. homatropine.
4. adrenaline.
5. cyclopentolate.

The contractile state of the iris muscles governs the size of the pupil. The outer radial muscles contract when their intrinsic nerves (sympathetic noradrenergic) are activated or when agonists act directly on the α-adrenoceptors of the muscle. The pupil then dilates. By contrast, the inner circular muscle contracts, leading to pupillary constriction, when the muscarinic cholinoceptors are stimulated either by drugs or through acetylcholine released from the cholinergic nerve supply. Since the circular muscle is normally partially contracted, drugs which inhibit parasympathetic function will cause pupillary dilatation. Such drugs will also reduce the pupillary light reflex since the narrowing of the pupil on exposure of the eye to bright light is brought about by the activation of parasympathetic fibres.

Atropinic drugs (e.g. **homatropine** or the shorter-acting **cyclopentolate**) will cause pupillary dilatation and will diminish the pupillary light reflex. **Atropine sulphate** is not used routinely in ophthalmology since its action may last for several days. In patients who are predisposed to narrow-angle glaucoma, atropinic drugs may precipitate an attack, especially if they are long-acting. However, **atropine** alternated with miotic agents has been used to prevent adhesions between the iris and lens in cases of iritis. **Adrenaline**, producing a weak transient dilatation of the pupil by stimulating the α-adrenoceptors on the radial muscle, will not prevent the circular muscle responding to bright light. **Cocaine** not only has a local anaesthetic activity, which would diminish the corneal blink reflex, but also is a potent inhibitor of the neuronal uptake of noradrenaline (uptake$_1$). By increasing the amounts of noradrenaline in the synaptic cleft and enhancing its actions, **cocaine** is sympathomimetic and causes pupil dilatation without the loss of the light reflex. By the same mechanism it causes vasoconstriction, leading to blanching of the conjunctiva. **Lignocaine** shares the local anaesthetic effects of **cocaine** but does not block uptake$_1$ and, therefore, the pupil is unaffected. With neither drug does the local anaesthesia extend into the iris as penetration through the aqueous humour is poor. Note that **cocaine** is approximately 1000 times more potent as an uptake blocker than as a local anaesthetic. FFTFT

Electrical stimulation of the intact cervical vagus nerve will

1. activate fibres from the carotid sinus baroreceptors.
2. promote gastric acid secretion.
3. cause a bradycardia resistant to **atropine**.
4. produce bronchospasm.
5. not affect the small intestine.

The paired vagus (tenth cranial nerve) is a mixed nerve, containing both afferent and efferent fibres all of which will be activated when the intact nerve is stimulated through an electrode placed on the cervical length. Impulses will travel along sensory nerves in the vagus to the CNS, where connections are made with sympathetic and parasympathetic efferent pathways. Baroreceptor afferents from the aortic arch run in the vagus but those from the carotid sinus run in the ninth cranial nerve (glossopharyngeal).

Impulses will also be conducted by the efferent fibres which innervate both thoracic and abdominal structures. Vagal efferent fibres carry the cranial parasympathetic outflow and are cholinergic nerves. When they are stimulated, bradycardia, bronchoconstriction, gastric acid secretion and contraction of the small intestine will all occur through the release of acetylcholine (ACh) from the postganglionic nerve terminals. Like all parasympathetic efferents, the vagus carries long preganglionic fibres terminating at the cell bodies of short postganglionic neurones embedded in the innervated tissue. Because ACh from preganglionic fibres acts through nicotinic receptors on the cell bodies, the effects of electrical stimulation can be reduced or abolished by nicotinic blockade. Thus **hexamethonium** or **mecamylamine** (drugs selective for these nicotinic receptors and therefore described as ganglion blockers) will inhibit vagal nerve stimulation.

The muscarinic receptor blocking drug **atropine** will also reduce the responses to electrical stimulation since all postganglionic parasympathetic fibres produce their effects via muscarinic receptors. However, these receptors have been subdivided into types M_1 and M_2 through the discovery of drugs with selective agonist or antagonist activity. **Pirenzipine** preferentially blocks M_1-receptors and is more effective in reducing the gastric acid secretion than in reducing the cardiac, bronchial or intestinal effects of vagal stimulation. High doses of **pirenzipine** will affect all these responses.

Using a variety of techniques, workers have demonstrated the coexistence of ACh and any of several peptides in some cholinergic nerves, especially in the intestine. Experiments have been described, particularly *in vitro*, in which responses of the viscera (e.g. gut or bladder contraction) to parasympathetic nerve stimulation have been resistant to **atropine**. A likely explanation is that simultaneously released peptides play an important part in the generation of these responses. FTFTF

MCQ 57

The cardiovascular effects of efferent vagal nerve stimulation and of a low dose of acetylcholine *injected intravenously*

1. are similar in that both cause a fall in peripheral resistance.
2. differ because only nerve stimulation will cause a significant bradycardia.
3. are abolished by **hexamethonium**.
4. differ in that **atropine** will block injected **acetylcholine** only.
5. will be potentiated by **physostigmine**.

The distribution and hence the principal effects of injected **acetylcholine** (**ACh**) and neuronally released acetylcholine (ACh) are different. Because ACh liberated from vagal nerves is hydrolysed very rapidly by acetylcholinesterase, little if any escapes from the synaptic cleft. Since blood vessels are not innervated by the vagus, they will not respond to vagal stimulation. Thus peripheral resistance does not change. Vessels will dilate in response to injected **ACh** since they possess muscarinic receptors. The sinoatrial node is relatively insensitive to concentrations of circulating **ACh** which are sufficient to cause vasodilatation. Therefore little change in heart rate will be produced by injected **ACh**.

Physostigmine inhibits all forms of cholinesterase and so preserves and thus potentiates both endogenous ACh and exogenous **ACh**. Since both cardiac and smooth muscle respond to **ACh** through a muscarinic mechanism, then no matter what the source of **ACh**, its actions will be prevented by the muscarinic blocking drug **atropine**. **Acetylcholine** causes vasodilatation through a complex mechanism which requires the presence of an intact endothelium. Stimulation of muscarinic receptors on the endothelial cells triggers the release of a vasodilator substance (endothelium-derived relaxing factor (EDRF), now thought to be nitric oxide). This material relaxes vascular smooth muscle by activating guanylate cyclase and thereby raising intracellular levels of cyclic GMP. The vasodilatation caused by, for example **bradykinin** is also considered to be due, at least in part, to the liberation of EDRF but, since this effect of **bradykinin** is not brought about through muscarinic receptors, it is unaffected by **atropine**.

Finally, only the responses caused by stimulation of the vagus involve nicotinic receptors (in the intervening ganglia). These will be blocked by **hexamethonium**, which probably acts by blocking sodium channels associated with the receptor. **Hexamethonium** is a member of the chemical series known as the polymethylene bisquaternary ammonium compounds. As its name suggests it possesses six methylene ($-CH_2-$) groups ($n = 6$), separating two quaternary nitrogen atoms:

$$(CH_3)_3N^+(CH_2)_nN^+(CH_3)_3$$

Another member, **pentamethonium** ($n = 5$), is also a ganglion blocker and another, **decamethonium** ($n = 10$), shows selectivity for the nicotinic receptors in skeletal muscle, where it is a partial agonist. FTFFT

The guinea-pig isolated ileum preparation

1. may be used to assess ganglion blocking activity.
2. exposed to **nicotine** will become refractory to **acetylcholine**.
3. will contract to **succinylcholine**.
4. will not respond to **dimethylphenylpiperazinium** after **atropine**.
5. exposed to **noradrenaline** will be less sensitive to **acetylcholine**.

The smooth muscle of the guinea-pig ileum is innervated by short postganglionic parasympathetic fibres whose cell bodies are found lying between longitudinal and circular muscle layers (Auerbach's plexus) and between the circular muscle layer and the mucosal cells (Meissner's plexus). Muscarinic cholinoceptors on the muscle cells mediate the spasmogenic action of acetylcholine (ACh) released from the postganglionic fibres, while nicotinic receptors on neuronal cell bodies mediate cholinergic ganglionic transmission. Thus **nicotine** and **dimethylphenylpiperazinium**, both of which stimulate nicotinic receptors, cause contraction because they promote the release of ACh from the postganglionic nerve endings onto muscarinic receptors on smooth muscle. Ganglion blocking drugs can, therefore, be assessed against these ganglion stimulants. Note, however, that atropinic agents, by acting on the smooth muscle, will also reduce the response to ganglion stimulants. It is usual, therefore, to demonstrate that the material assessed as a ganglion blocker does not affect the response to exogenous **ACh** (i.e. does not have muscarinic blocking properties).

Added **ACh** will act primarily on the smooth muscle muscarinic receptors, which are not affected directly by **nicotine**. **Succinylcholine** (a partial agonist at nicotinic receptors of skeletal muscle) in concentrations effective at the neuromuscular junction does not stimulate the ganglionic receptors, which are not identical to the nicotinic receptors in skeletal muscle.

Adrenoceptors, both α- and β-, are found in the ileum. α_2-Adrenoceptors are mainly on cholinergic neurones and their stimulation will inhibit ACh release. α- and β-adrenoceptors are found postsynaptically (on muscle fibres) and their stimulation leads to muscular relaxation. Thus **noradrenaline**, which can stimulate both types of adrenoceptor, is a functional antagonist of **ACh**.

Because the guinea-pig isolated ileum is usually in a completely relaxed state, drugs can only be assessed through their ability to cause contraction or to modify the contractions induced by other means. Intestinal segments from species like mouse or rabbit exhibit rhythmic pendular movements and are in a state of partial contraction even in the absence of drugs. Therefore, in such preparations, functional antagonists (e.g. sympathomimetic drugs, methylxanthines) are seen directly to cause muscle relaxation and inhibition of the pendular movements. TFFTT

MCQ 59

Both guanethidine *and* hexamethonium *will block responses of the*

1. guinea-pig vas deferens to stimulation through the hypogastric nerve.
2. coaxially stimulated guinea-pig ileum preparation.
3. Finkleman preparation of rabbit ileum stimulated through its periarterial nerves.
4. phrenic nerve–diaphragm preparation to stimulation of the phrenic nerve.
5. vas deferens to transmural stimulation.

Guanethidine is an adrenergic neurone blocking drug used in the treatment of severe hypertension, while **hexamethonium** is a ganglion blocking drug with little clinical use. For *both* to be effective in an isolated preparation, stimulation must be applied *preganglionically* to *noradrenergic* nerves.

The vas deferens receives a sympathetic motor innervation which is largely noradrenergic through the hypogastric nerve, though there may be other transmitters involved in addition. Atypically, the hypogastric nerve contains ganglia which have been found as near as 1–2 mm from the organ. Stimulation by electrodes on the nerve will, therefore, be blocked by both drugs. Transmural (i.e. field) stimulation produces a response mediated through the excitation of postganglionic fibres and so **hexamethonium** is ineffective.

By contrast with the vas deferens, the sympathetic postganglionic fibres to the gut are long. In the Finkleman preparation these fibres are stimulated as they run along the mesenteric arteries (periarterially) and so the relaxation of the gut produced by stimulation is unaffected by **hexamethonium**.

Coaxial stimulation is similar to transmural or field stimulation and causes contractions of the guinea-pig ileum mediated through parasympathetic postganglionic cholinergic fibres, which are unaffected by **hexamethonium** or **guanethidine**.

The diaphragm is a skeletal muscle and its phrenic nerve is somatic. The nicotinic receptors are, therefore, little affected by **hexamethonium** and the cholinergic transmission is not blocked by **guanethidine**.

There is increasing evidence that peripheral nerves use a variety of neurochemicals besides acetylcholine (ACh) and noradrenaline to regulate the functions of innervated cells. In some cases separate fibres exist, for example in gut plexuses, which liberate neurotransmitters such as 5-hydroxytryptamine; in others, additional substances, such as peptides and purines, coexist with the classical neurotransmitters. Since field stimulation of isolated organs stimulates all neurones present, the response of the organs is the sum of the effects of all the liberated materials. Thus, for example, the resistance to blockade by **atropine** of bladder contractions to parasympathetic nerve stimulation may be explained by the actions of neurochemicals other than ACh. TFFFF

A drug reduced the effect of vagal nerve stimulation in the isolated right atrium but did not affect the basal rate of beat. It can be correctly concluded that the drug

1. is a muscarinic receptor blocker.
2. is a ganglion blocker.
3. does not affect noradrenergic neurotransmission.
4. would block the response to added **acetylcholine**.
5. would also reduce responses of the diaphragm to stimulation of the phrenic nerve.

The right atrium contains the pacemaker tissue of the sinoatrial (SA) node, where the beat of the intact heart originates. Under suitable conditions of temperature and oxygenation the SA node will cause spontaneous coordinated atrial beats in isolated tissue. In an isolated atrium the rate of beating will be determined by the inherent activity of the SA node because the intrinsic nerves are quiescent. However, the nodal cells possess both muscarinic cholinoceptors and β_1-adrenoceptors, which are accessible to autonomic neurotransmitters or to exogenous drugs which may interact with these receptors and alter the rate of beating.

There are several types of drug activity which would explain the observed effects, but none of the alternatives in the question is conclusively demonstrated without further evidence. For instance, a muscarinic receptor blocking drug, like **atropine**, would produce the required effects (and would block the response to added **acetylcholine**). A ganglion blocker, like **hexamethonium**, would also produce the desired effects (since there are ganglia in the vagal pathway) but would not block the actions of added **acetylcholine**. Thus either is possible and more evidence is required if these two alternatives are to be distinguished. It could be correctly concluded that the drug was *not* an agonist *in the concentration(s) used* at either muscarinic cholinoceptors or β_1-adrenoceptors since a decrease or an increase respectively in basal rate would have occurred. This conclusion illustrates that negative results can be just as meaningful as positives in the interpretation of experiments.

From the results of this limited experiment on atrial muscle it is impossible to predict the actions of the drug on a diaphragm preparation. Not only are the end-organs different (cardiac pacemaker and skeletal muscle respectively) but so are their types of receptor (muscarinic/β_1-adrenoceptor and nicotinic respectively); their only similarity is in the nature of the stimulated nerves, i.e. cholinergic in each case.

It is vitally important to appreciate that, just because a particular hypothesis may explain an experimental result, it should not be taken as correct until alternative explanations have been disproved. FFFFF

Peripheral Noradrenergic Nervous System

Sympathetic postganglionic fibres which synthesize noradrenaline

1. are properly termed adrenergic.
2. synthesize dopa through a rate-limiting step from tyrosine.
3. may be depleted of their transmitter if tyrosine hydroxylase is inhibited.
4. do not synthesize dopa in the presence of **α-methyldopa**.
5. will not release transmitter when stimulated in the presence of **disulphiram**.

Sympathetic postganglionic nerve fibres are loosely termed 'adrenergic' because they were originally thought to release adrenaline. The more correct term, 'noradrenergic', should be used and the term 'adrenergic' restricted to some CNS neurones and to amphibian sympathetic fibres where adrenaline is the neurotransmitter. A few sympathetic nerves, such as those to the sweat glands, are cholinergic but are the exception to the rule.

The biosynthesis of noradrenaline (NA) starts when tyrosine is taken up into the nerve and converted to the catechol derivative dopa (dihydroxyphenylalanine) by tyrosine hydroxylase. This reaction is the rate-limiting step in the pathway so the level of enzyme activity critically affects the production of neurotransmitter. A negative feedback mechanism exists where the endproduct of the synthesis (NA) inhibits the activity of the enzyme through competition with an essential pteridine co-factor. A slower trans-synaptic regulation also occurs where high levels of neuronal activity cause increased synthesis of the enzyme. **α-Methyl-*p*-tyrosine** is an inhibitor of this enzyme and when given *in vivo* reduces NA synthesis, leading to eventual transmitter depletion.

Dopa is converted to dopamine by aromatic L-amino acid decarboxylase (also found in 5-hydroxytryptamine-containing nerves), which can be blocked by **α-methyldopa**. Large doses of this drug will reduce the store of NA in the nerve, but the total store of amines is little affected since **α-methyldopa** is biotransformed and the α-methyl derivatives simply replace the normal amines.

Dopamine is transported across the membrane of the storage granule by a carrier system. Within the granule, dopamine β-hydroxylase converts dopamine to NA, which is then stored as a complex with ATP and specialized proteins (chromogranins). Dopamine β-hydroxylase can be blocked by **fusaric acid** and **disulphiram**, but little reduction occurs in transmitter levels since this is not the rate-limiting step in the synthesis. In addition to its precursor role, dopamine is known to be a neurotransmitter in its own right, both in several CNS pathways and in the periphery (e.g. kidney and coronary vascular beds).

Adrenergic nerves (and the cells of the adrenal medulla) possess an enzyme (phenylethanolamine *N*-methyltransferase; PNMT) which methylates the amino group, changing the primary amine NA into the secondary amine adrenaline. The presence of this enzyme is essential if the nerve is to be correctly termed adrenergic.

The coexistence in many nerves of amines with either purines or peptides has led to the suggestion that these neurochemicals have co-transmitter or modulator functions. FTTFF

MCQ 62

Termination of the effects of endogenous noradrenaline

1. is faster when monoamine oxidase is blocked.
2. occurs mainly by uptake of the amine into non-neuronal cells.
3. takes longer in the presence of **cocaine**.
4. occurs almost exclusively in the liver.
5. is only important in experiments on whole animals.

Noradrenaline (NA) released from sympathetic nerves may act at several types of receptor located on pre- or postsynaptic membranes. To prevent excessive stimulation of these receptors, NA must be quickly removed from their vicinity. Although the enzymes monoamine oxidase (MAO) and catechol-*O*-methyltransferase (COMT) destroy NA, other processes are mainly responsible for this removal. Principally, a transport process (uptake$_1$) carries extracellular NA through the axonal membrane and thereby removes about 80% of the NA from the synaptic cleft. The uptake$_1$ process is active (energy requiring), shows stereoselectivity, (−)-NA being transported much more effectively than (+)-NA, and can be blocked by tricyclic antidepressants, like **desmethylimipramine**, or by **cocaine** (which has an additional local anaesthetic effect at higher concentrations). Uptake blocking drugs may enhance the response to NA since a higher concentration remains in the locality of the receptors.

Paradoxically, the actions of *indirectly* acting sympathomimetic amines like **tyramine** are reduced by uptake$_1$ blockade since they must enter the nerve via this transport system before displacing NA from its storage sites to produce their indirect effects.

Noradrenaline enters non-neuronal cells by the uptake$_2$ process, which is not stereoselective, has a lower affinity for NA and is blocked by drugs such as **17-β-oestradiol**, corticosteroids and the NA metabolite **normetanephrine**. Some drugs (e.g. **isoprenaline**) are avidly taken up by the uptake$_2$ process but are not transported by uptake$_1$.

The uptake processes affect NA in three ways: first, by removing it from the synaptic cleft and curtailing its actions; second, by transporting it into the nerve, where it may be used again; third, by transporting NA into the locality of the metabolizing enzymes MAO and COMT.

Monoamine oxidase exists in two major isomeric forms (types A and B), differing in substrate specificity and in the selectivity of inhibitors towards them. Both types are found in brain and in liver; human placenta has only type A and platelets only type B. Many amines are biotransformed by MAO: for instance, NA is a preferred substrate for type A, while **tyramine** is biotransformed by both types, being rapidly deaminated in gut, liver and nerve cells. In the presence of MAO inhibitors (like the non-selective **pargyline**) foods containing **tyramine** (some wines, cheeses, yeast extracts) are dangerous because preserving the amine leads to enhancement of its indirect sympathomimetic actions. The effects of NA are less obviously affected by inhibitors since removal of NA from its site of action is mainly by other means.   FFTFF

Depletion of tissue stores of noradrenaline

1. can be produced by section of preganglionic sympathetic nerves.
2. occurs on treatment with **reserpine**, which also affects stores of 5-hydroxytryptamine.
3. when caused by sympathetic ganglionectomy can be restored by infusion of **noradrenaline**.
4. occurs when **6-hydroxydopamine** is used to destroy noradrenergic nerves.
5. may be caused by **guanethidine**.

The storage and release of noradrenaline (NA) from noradrenergic nerves is subject to many controlling mechanisms. Intraneuronal NA can inhibit both tyrosine hydroxylase and dopamine β-oxidase, thereby inhibiting its own synthesis. These mechanisms account for the remarkably constant levels of NA which are normally found in any given tissue, though large differences in absolute levels occur between different organs (e.g. vas deferens, heart and intestine contain 15, 1.5 and 0.5 μg NA per gram of tissue respectively).

Reserpine depletes nerves of their NA content (and acts similarly on nerves containing dopamine or 5-hydroxytryptamine). Its action is on the membrane of the storage granule, in low concentrations to prevent the transport of NA and dopamine and in high concentrations to cause the membrane to leak the granule contents into the cytoplasm. Most of the cytoplasmic amines would then be deaminated by mitochondrial monoamine oxidase but at very high doses of **reserpine** some amines could escape from the neurone, producing sympathomimetic effects. **Reserpine** crosses the blood–brain barrier and depletes CNS neurones of their monoamine transmitters. This is responsible for the neuroleptic, depressant and, in part, the antihypertensive effects of **reserpine**.

Any agent damaging nerve fibres can cause loss of transmitter and depletion of tissue stores. This can occur with (a) **6-hydroxydopamine**, which is taken up by uptake$_1$, concentrated in the nerve and biotransformed to a neurotoxic peroxide; (b) **nerve growth factor antiserum**, which combines immunologically with and inactivates nerve growth factor, which is essential to the development of sympathetic nerves; and (c) surgical section of the nerves, causing the peripheral portion to degenerate slowly. Section of *pre*ganglionic fibres does not affect the storage of NA in postganglionic neurones.

The specificity of these methods varies. For example, dopaminergic and noradrenergic nerves may be destroyed by **6-hydroxydopamine**, which is sometimes injected into discrete brain areas. **Nerve growth factor antiserum** works only in very young animals (and optimally in rats and mice) and normally affects only the undeveloped efferent sympathetic nerves.

Guanethidine, an adrenergic neurone blocker, depletes tissues of NA and this effect is separate from the adrenergic neurone blockade which is seen before gross changes in NA content take place. In high doses **guanethidine** may cause some destruction of noradrenergic nerves and attempts have been made to use this action to produce sympathectomy in animals.   FTFTT

MCQ 64

Adrenoceptors found in sympathetically innervated tissues

1. are preferentially stimulated by **clonidine** if they belong to the α_2-subgroup.
2. are principally of the β_1-subgroup when located postsynaptically in the heart.
3. if belonging to the α_2-subgroup, are involved in a feedback mechanism to increase noradrenaline release when stimulated.
4. are preferentially blocked by **prazosin** if they belong to the α_1-subgroup.
5. if presynaptic, can only be detected by measuring neurotransmitter release.

Receptors on which neurotransmitters act exist not only postsynaptically but also presynaptically on the membrane of the nerve itself. Noradrenergic nerves have presynaptic α-adrenoceptors which appear to control the amounts of noradrenaline (NA) released. They are involved in a negative feedback mechanism whereby released NA can inhibit the further release of NA. Drug effectiveness at these receptors is usually assessed by measuring the amounts of NA released by electrical stimulation at frequencies of 1–10 Hz. Alternatively, the tissues can be incubated with radiolabelled NA, which is taken up into the stores. Stimulation then releases radiolabelled transmitter, which can be measured easily in terms of the amounts of radioactivity produced. However, presynaptic actions of drugs can also be detected by responses of the end-organ since, other things being equal, increased transmitter release will evoke a larger response and vice versa. Care is needed in interpreting such responses because factors in addition to amounts released are important (e.g. uptake processes, drug selectivity).

α-Adrenoceptor blockers such as **phentolamine** and **phenoxybenzamine** cause more NA to be liberated per pulse; agonists like **NA** itself or **clonidine** may stimulate the presynaptic receptors and reduce transmitter release. These findings explain why some α-adrenoceptor blockers such as **phentolamine** are less effective in blocking the effects of nerve stimulation than they are at blocking exogenous **NA**. **Phentolamine** not only reduces the effectiveness of **NA** on receptors in the end-organ (e.g. smooth muscle) but also simultaneously increases the amounts of NA released from nerves by its blocking action on presynaptic receptors.

Analysis of the affinities of several agonists and antagonists for the pre- and postsynaptic receptors has shown that the bulk of the receptors are not identical in these two locations. The term α_2 is now used to describe the type of receptor mainly involved in the control of NA release, while α_1 is used to describe the type which mainly mediates the response to NA postsynaptically. Drugs which show some selectivity between these receptor types are: *agonists,* α_2: **clonidine, oxymetazoline, naphazoline;** α_1: **methoxamine, phenylephrine;** *antagonists,* α_2: **yohimbine, idazoxan;** α_1: **clozapine, prazosin.**

Finally, it should be noted that stimulation of presynaptic β-adrenoceptors may facilitate NA release and that a variety of other presynaptic receptors are present on the nerve terminals (reacting to acetylcholine, dopamine, histamine, opioids and prostaglandins among others). TTFTF

Adrenoceptors

1. are classified as β_2 when their blockade leads to bronchodilatation.
2. were designated α and β by Ahlquist on the basis of the relative activity of a series of agonists.
3. in the iris, causing pupillary dilatation, are of the α_1-subgroup.
4. of the α_2-type are stimulated by **noradrenaline**.
5. of both the α- and β-types mediate intestinal relaxation.

Noradrenaline causes its effects by interacting with adrenoceptors located on the membranes of the effector cells. Several distinct types of receptors are recognized. They differ in their selectivity for agonists and antagonists and in their anatomical location. A division into α- and β-adrenoceptors to explain variations in the responsiveness of different organs to several sympathomimetics was first proposed by Alhquist in 1948. His proposals predicted the discovery of drugs which could block the β-adrenoceptors (β-adrenoceptor stimulants as well as both agonists and antagonists at the α-site were already known). The development of more drugs acting on β-adrenoceptors led to the recognition by 1964 that differences between the actions of some of them could be explained if β-adrenoceptors were not a homogeneous group but were divided into β_1- and β_2-types. In a similar fashion, about 10 years later, the α-adrenoceptors were divided into α_1- and α_2-types.

β_1-Adrenoceptors are responsible principally for increasing the rate and force of the heart beat and for stimulating lipolysis in fat cells. Most other functions of β-adrenoceptors are inhibitory (e.g. bronchodilatation and vasodilatation, intestinal muscle relaxation) though some are excitatory (e.g. raising blood sugar). **Isoprenaline** stimulates both β_1- and β_2-adrenoceptors. **Noradrenaline** stimulates β_1-adrenoceptors but has little effect on those of the β_2-type. **Salbutamol** is much more effective on the β_2- than the β_1-type.

The α-adrenoceptors found postsynaptically in almost every organ receiving sympathetic nerves are generally excitatory and belong mainly to the α_1-subgroup. Thus vasoconstriction and contraction of the smooth muscle of vas deferens and spleen occur through α_1-adrenoceptor stimulation. The receptor found on noradrenergic and other nerve terminals is mainly the α_2-type, stimulation of which causes a reduction in transmitter release. In addition, α_2-adrenoceptors are found postsynaptically, where they mediate smooth muscle contraction. For instance, in some blood vessels, α_2-adrenoceptors are located on the muscle in positions further away from noradrenergic nerve endings than the α_1-receptors, which has led to the suggestion that these α_2-adrenoceptors may be activated principally by circulating catecholamines. Paradoxically, α- as well as β-adrenoceptors are involved in intestinal relaxation; both classes are present on the muscle cells, although a component of the relaxation is due to stimulation of presynaptic α_2-adrenoceptors, which inhibits release of excitatory neurotransmitters such as acetylcholine. **Noradrenaline** stimulates both α_1- and α_2-, **phenylephrine** is selective towards α_1-, and **clonidine** towards α_2-adrenoceptors. FTTTT

MCQ 66

The adenylate cyclase/cyclic AMP system is activated by

1. β-adrenoceptors in the heart.
2. β-adrenoceptors in the liver.
3. nicotinic cholinoceptors at the neuromuscular junction.
4. histamine H₂-receptors in the heart.
5. **cholera toxin**.

Transmembrane signalling (the conversion of the extracellular action of an agonist into a change in intracellular activity) can be achieved by receptor-operated ion channels or by a second messenger system.

One receptor-operated ion channel involves nicotinic receptors at the skeletal muscle end-plate, where protein subunits (β, γ, δ and two α) span the membrane, forming an ion channel. **Acetylcholine** interacts with the α-subunits of the nicotinic receptor to open the ion channel, allowing sodium to enter. If the resulting end-plate depolarization is sufficient, then *voltage-* (potential-) operated sodium channels in the muscle membrane will pass a conducted action potential across the muscle surface, initiating contraction. Note the distinction between *receptor*-operated (agonist-sensitive) and *voltage*-operated ion channels.

The adenylate cyclase/cyclic AMP system and the phosphoinositide system form two second messenger systems and there are many similarities in their detailed operation. In each, an enzyme (adenylate cyclase and phospholipase C respectively) is linked to receptor(s), activation of which modulates the enzyme activity. In the cardiac cyclic AMP system, histamine H₂-receptors and β-adrenoceptors are both linked to adenylate cyclase. The β-adrenoceptor is a protein which has seven segments spanning the membrane. The face presented to the extracellular environment binds to the β-adrenoceptor agonist (e.g. **isoprenaline**) and this induces changes in the tertiary structure of the transmembrane segments or in the protein linkage joining the transmembrane segments on the cytoplasmic side. This change allows the inner part of the receptor to bind to a regulatory unit, the G protein, which then binds GTP. The G protein–GTP complex binds in turn to adenylate cyclase and activates it to transform ATP into cyclic AMP. The GTP is then hydrolysed by GTPase, allowing the G protein to dissociate from adenylate cyclase, which returns to its former unactivated state. In this way the extracellular combination of an agonist with its receptor produces a rise in intracellular levels of cyclic AMP. **Cholera toxin** binds to the GTPase and so prevents the hydrolysis of GTP; the complex remains attached to adenylate cyclase, which is held in an active state.

The rise in intracellular cyclic AMP levels activates a cyclic AMP-dependent protein kinase which is able to phosphorylate various enzymes and modify their activity. Thus in liver a lipase is activated, as is phosphorylase kinase, which in turn activates phosphorylase A – hence the increased lipolysis (rise in free fatty acids) and increased breakdown of glycogen (rise in blood glucose) following β-adrenoceptor stimulation. Glycogen synthetase is also phosphorylated but this *decreases* its activity, causing a reduction in the rate of glycogen synthesis which contributes to the rise in blood glucose. TTFTT

The second messenger phosphoinositide system is activated by

1. γ-aminobutyric acid receptors in the CNS.
2. muscarinic receptors in salivary gland.
3. protein kinase C.
4. phospholipase C.
5. phospholipase A_2.

Transmembrane signalling (conversion of the extracellular action of an agonist into a change in intracellular activity) can be achieved by receptor-operated ion channels or by the action of second messenger systems.

One receptor-operated ion channel involves γ-aminobutyric acid (GABA) receptors of the $GABA_A$ type, which are linked to the chloride channel. When GABA acts on these receptors, the chloride channel is opened and chloride ions flow into the cell, cause hyperpolarization and inhibit cell firing. Hence the classification of GABA as an inhibitory transmitter. Note that some ion channels (voltage-sensitive) are not triggered by receptors but are operated by changes in membrane potential (e.g. the sodium channel in neurones). Thus an agonist may open a receptor-operated ion channel and cause depolarization of the cell membrane; this may in turn open a voltage-operated channel to allow ion movements which may reinforce or oppose the original change in potential.

The adenylate cyclase/cyclic AMP system and the phosphoinositide system are both second messenger systems. In the heart the former is linked to β-adrenoceptors, to histamine H_2-receptors and to glucagon receptors and activation of any of these will cause inotropic and chronotropic responses associated with a rise in intracellular cyclic AMP concentration.

By contrast, other agonists (e.g. acetylcholine on muscarinic receptors in salivary gland or noradrenaline on some $α_1$-adrenoceptors) activate receptors linked to phospholipase C (probably through similar G proteins as were discovered in the cyclic AMP system). Activation of phospholipase C causes inositol-4,5-diphosphate to be transformed to two materials: triphosphoinositol (inositol-1,4,5-triphosphate) and diacylglycerol (DAG). The former is released into the cytosol and can cause release of calcium from intracellular binding sites. The free calcium ion concentration in the cytoplasm is normally maintained below about 10^{-7} M in a resting cell but on liberation of the ion from intracellular stores (or inflow through the membrane from extracellular fluid) free calcium concentration rises and calcium combines with its binding protein calmodulin. This protein is involved in most of the intracellular effects of calcium and each molecule can bind up to four calcium ions, the number being related to the intracellular calcium concentration. The calmodulin–calcium complex can affect membranes both by altering permeability to ions and by influencing exocytosis and can also activate various enzymes, for example some protein kinases, calcium-activated ATPase, guanylate cyclase and phospholipase A_2. This last enzyme is responsible for generating arachidonic acid from membrane phospholipids (hence leading to prostaglandins, leukotrienes and platelet activating factor).

continued on next page

On the other hand, DAG activates membrane-bound protein kinase C, which can phosphorylate proteins and therefore control activity of many enzymes, promoting a variety of responses (e.g. platelet aggregation). Diacylglycerol lipase converts DAG to glycerol and arachidonic acid, a further source of prostaglandins and leukotrienes.   FTFTF

An example of the mechanism by which a substance brings about its pharmacological effect is

1. **17-β-oestradiol** through the cyclic AMP system.
2. **insulin** through receptor-operated ion channels.
3. **pertussis toxin** through the cyclic AMP system.
4. **forskolin** through receptor-operated ion channels.
5. **theophylline** through the cyclic AMP system.

Insulin, a large protein which cannot diffuse easily into cells, combines with its receptor on the cell membranes. The receptor consists of an α-unit to which insulin binds and a transmembrane β-component. The sequence of events leading to **insulin**'s actions (alterations in glucose carriers, increased glycolysis and decreased glycogenolysis etc.) is unclear but may involve production of peptide mediators or activation of protein kinases. However, receptor-operated ion channels are not thought to be involved.

A variety of membrane receptors (e.g. β-adrenoceptors) are linked through stimulatory G proteins to adenylate cyclase, which catalyses the conversion of ATP to cyclic AMP. Intracellular levels of cyclic AMP will therefore rise when these receptors are stimulated. However, cyclic AMP can also be generated by substances which bypass the receptor and act through either the G proteins (e.g. **cholera toxin, fluoride** ions) or on adenylate cyclase itself (e.g. **forskolin**). By contrast, other G proteins exist which exert an *inhibitory* action on adenylate cyclase; receptors linked to these are said to be negatively coupled to the enzyme. A protein (**pertussis toxin**) in whooping cough vaccine combines with the *inhibitory* G protein, locking it in an inactive state, and thereby prevents receptor-mediated inhibition of adenylate cyclase. Thus, in cells where this inhibitory system has an important suppressive role, **pertussis toxin** would be expected to raise the levels of cyclic AMP. A further mechanism by which cyclic AMP could be elevated is by blocking the enzymes (phosphodiesterases) which break down the nucleotide. **Theophylline**, a methylxanthine which is a phosphodiesterase inhibitor, permits an accumulation of cyclic AMP in cells and potentiates the effects of substances which act by increasing cyclic AMP production.

Unlike large molecules such as **insulin**, steroid hormones are not generally confined to the extracellular space but, because of their high lipid solubility, penetrate cells; this permits a direct action on intracellular receptors though several hours may elapse before their effects are expressed. Oestrogens (e.g. **17-β-oestradiol**) affect principally the vagina, uterus, mammary glands and certain tumours because these target tissues possess many oestrogen-binding molecules in the cytoplasm. After binding, the oestrogen–receptor complex is translocated to the nucleus, where RNA and protein synthesis is initiated. If the complex is maintained in the nucleus, DNA synthesis may also be initiated. The antioestrogen **tamoxifen** binds to the oestrogen receptors, fails to activate protein synthesis and prevents oestrogenic actions; it can therefore be used in the treatment of oestrogen-dependent mammary carcinomas.   FFTFT

MCQ 69

Drugs with sympathomimetic properties

1. are mostly catecholamines like **adrenaline** and **phenylephrine**.
2. may have no efficacy on adrenoceptors.
3. like **dopamine** may be used to treat cardiogenic shock.
4. may be used as nasal decongestants if their principal action is on β-adrenoceptors.
5. by stimulating β_2-adrenoceptors may reduce the release of substances from mast cells in an asthmatic attack.

The term 'sympathomimetic' describes any drug which, interacting with adrenoceptors or neurones, produces effects resembling those caused by stimulation of sympathetic nerves. Therefore **adrenaline**, **isoprenaline**, **phenylephrine** and **salbutamol** are all sympathomimetics. **Adrenaline** and **isoprenaline** are also catecholamines, i.e. they have a phenyl ring possessing two adjacent hydroxyl substituents, but the other two are not.

Drugs which stimulate β-adrenoceptors in preference to α-receptors (and therefore stimulate the heart and relax vascular, uterine and bronchiolar muscles) have a major use as bronchodilators in hay fever and asthma. In these respiratory disorders it is desirable to have as little cardiac stimulation as possible, so drugs like **salbutamol**, **terbutaline** and **rimiterol** which show selectivity towards β_2-adrenoceptors are often preferred. They also stimulate β_2-adrenoceptors on mast cells, raising cyclic AMP levels, which stabilizes the mast cell membrane and inhibits histamine release.

Cardiac arrest and complete heart block may be treated with β_1-stimulants. Cardiogenic shock may be treated with **dobutamine**, a β_1-agonist, or **dopamine**, which stimulates β_1- as well as dopamine receptors. In low doses both drugs increase cardiac output but produce little vasoconstriction.

Drugs which stimulate α-adrenoceptors in preference to β-adrenoceptors are used to produce vasoconstriction or to dilate the pupil. **Adrenaline** is added to local anaesthetic solutions to delay removal of the anaesthetic from the site of administration and thus prolong the action. **Phenylephrine** and other similar agents are used as nasal decongestants (by constricting nasal blood vessels) in hay-fever attacks. Given as eye-drops, **adrenaline** and **phenylephrine** cause mydriasis (by contraction of the dilator pupillae muscles) and reduce conjunctival hyperaemia. As mydriatics they may be preferred to atropinic drugs as they do not interfere with accommodation and do not precipitate glaucoma. Instead, they may reduce intraocular pressure by reducing the rate of formation of the aqueous humour.

Other sympathomimetics act indirectly. **Tyramine** and **amphetamine** enter noradrenergic nerves and displace noradrenaline (NA), which produces the biological effects. **Cocaine** is sympathomimetic both by releasing NA and by preventing its reuptake into nerves (uptake$_1$), thus preserving a higher concentration in the vicinity of the receptors. **Cocaine** itself does not activate adrenoceptors, though high concentrations of **tyramine** and **amphetamine** can do so.   FTTFT

If injected intravenously into an anaesthetized cat

1. both **clonidine** and **phenylephrine** would initially raise diastolic pressure.
2. neither **salbutamol** nor **isoprenaline** would cause bradycardia.
3. **isoprenaline** would increase the pulse pressure by stimulating cardiac ventricular β_1-adrenoceptors.
4. **phenylephrine** may cause bradycardia by stimulating muscarinic receptors at the sinoatrial node.
5. both **phenylephrine** and **salbutamol** would dilate blood vessels in skeletal muscle.

The effects of agonists and antagonists at adrenoceptors can be predicted from a knowledge of the receptor distribution and of sympathetic nervous system function. For instance, **phenylephrine** is a selective stimulant of α_1-adrenoceptors. Given i.v., it will raise the blood pressure by causing vasoconstriction, whilst heart rate will probably fall through reflex activity, initiated by the pressor response. Administered locally or to isolated tissues, it will dilate the pupil (by contracting the radial muscle of the iris) and contract the sphincters in the gut and other smooth muscle generally.

The agonist actions of **clonidine** (selective towards α_2-adrenoceptors) are best revealed on isolated tissues during electrical stimulation of the sympathetic nerves. **Clonidine** reduces responses to nerve stimulation by diminishing the amounts of noradrenaline (NA) released per nerve impulse. It activates the autoinhibitory mechanism mediated through presynaptic α_2-adrenoceptors, by which NA can diminish its own release. Given i.v., **clonidine** causes a transient pressor effect by stimulating α_1-adrenoceptors on vascular smooth muscle. It causes both bradycardia and hypotension by increasing vagal and decreasing sympathetic activity through an action on the α_2-adrenoceptors in the CNS.

Isoprenaline causes a fall in diastolic blood pressure through stimulation of vasodilator β_2-adrenoceptors. Pulse pressure rises due to increased force of cardiac contraction which, like the simultaneous tachycardia, occurs through β_1 stimulation. The rise in pulse pressure means that the systolic level may be higher in spite of the diastolic fall, though there is usually an overall lowering of mean blood pressure after **isoprenaline**.

If tone in the smooth muscle of the respiratory tract is high, **isoprenaline** will cause bronchodilatation (β_2) but in some species (guinea-pig, rat) bronchoconstriction may have to be induced before this effect can be demonstrated. On isolated smooth muscle (gut, trachea, vas deferens) **isoprenaline** usually has relaxant effects if tone is high. With **salbutamol** (selective towards β_2-adrenoceptors) bronchodilatation and vasodilatation are produced at doses which have little effect on the heart. TTTFF

MCQ 71

When electrical stimulation of preganglionic sympathetic nerves causes a release of noradrenaline the

1. release can be prevented by **tubocurarine**.
2. release can be enhanced by **tetrodotoxin**.
3. noradrenaline will be largely transported back into the nerve.
4. release can be reduced by **guanethidine**.
5. replacement of the noradrenaline in the stores occurs mainly by synthesis of new noradrenaline.

The release of transmitter from noradrenergic nerves can be prevented by various drugs; which ones are effective may depend on how the nerve is excited. The effects of electrical stimulation of preganglionic fibres or of stimulation of the nicotinic receptors in ganglia by drugs such as **dimethylphenylpiperazinium (DMPP)** will both be inhibited by ganglion blockers such as **hexamethonium**. **Tubocurarine** is also a ganglion blocking agent in doses only slightly higher than are needed to block nicotinic receptors at the neuromuscular junction. Local anaesthetics, **tetrodotoxin** or cooling of the nerve will all stop noradrenaline (NA) release simply by preventing the conduction of the impulse to the nerve terminals, though this effect is not confined to noradrenergic nerves.

Adrenergic neurone blockers like **guanethidine** and **bretylium** enter the noradrenergic nerve via the uptake$_1$ process and their action can, therefore, be prevented by uptake-blocking drugs. Once inside they may interfere with the utilization of Ca^{2+} in excitation–secretion coupling or they may deplete a very small store of NA which is essential for neurotransmission.

Guanethidine given i.v. causes a sympathomimetic response by displacing NA from vesicles and may, in fact, enter vesicles since it can be released by electrical stimulation of tissues which have accumulated it. **Guanethidine** also acts as an uptake$_1$ blocker whilst occupying this transport mechanism and this contributes towards its ability to potentiate extracellular NA, though there is insufficient potentiation to offset significantly the adrenergic neurone blockade. Although other antihypertensive therapies have taken precedence, **guanethidine** is used to treat severe hypertension and acts to reduce vasoconstrictor tone. It has all the undesirable effects associated with loss of sympathetic tone (postural hypotension, diarrhoea, failure of ejaculation).

Although the majority of neurones in postganglionic sympathetic pathways are noradrenergic, a release of other substances which may have neurotransmitter or neuromodulatory functions has often been detected during nerve stimulation. Some of these (e.g. ATP, neuropeptide-Y) coexist in neurones with NA, although in certain cases they may exist in separate cells. It should be borne in mind that drugs which interfere with sympathetic function may do so by affecting the co-transmitter either alone or simultaneously with NA. Thus, in vas deferens, **guanethidine** blocks the release of both ATP and NA from electrically stimulated nerves; alternatively a combination of **prazosin** (an α_1-adrenoceptor blocker) and $\alpha\beta$-**methylene ATP** (a substance causing desensitization to ATP) is required to abolish completely the muscle contraction. TFTTF

Drugs that can reduce the vascular effects of sympathetic nerve stimulation

1. may act by blocking postsynaptic α-adrenoceptors.
2. may act by stimulating cardiac β-adrenoceptors.
3. include alkaloids like **dihydroergotamine**, which also causes uterine muscle contraction.
4. include **phenoxybenzamine**, which also blocks the uptake$_1$ mechanism transporting noradrenaline into the neuronal cytoplasm.
5. include **prazosin**, which is used in the treatment of hypertension.

The effects of noradrenergic nerve stimulation can be blocked by drugs acting on the nerve to prevent the release of noradrenaline (NA) or by drugs blocking the postsynaptic receptors. Thus α_1-adrenoceptor blockers will prevent NA from contracting smooth muscle. β-Adrenoceptor blockers will prevent the cardiac (β_1) effects and the actions of sympathomimetics in relaxing vascular and bronchial smooth muscle (β_2).

Early in the 20th century, Dale and his co-workers isolated several biologically active alkaloids from the fungus ergot, which contaminates the cereal crop rye. Some of the amino-acid-containing alkaloids and their semisynthetic derivatives (e.g. **dihydroergotamine**) were shown to antagonize the pressor effect of i.v. **adrenaline** in the cat. These drugs were the first α-adrenoceptor blockers to be discovered, although they were not named as such for a further 40 years. However, **ergotamine** has additional pharmacological effects producing, for instance, vasoconstriction and uterine contractions (for which reason it should be avoided in pregnancy). It also promotes nausea and vomiting, probably by stimulating the chemoreceptor trigger zone in the medullary vomiting centre. **Dihydroergotamine**, by contrast, is inactive on the uterus and is a less potent vasoconstrictor. **Ergotamine**, by mouth, is used to relieve migraine, as is occasionally **dihydroergotamine**, given i.m. Their precise mode of action is unknown, though it probably involves interference with 5-hydroxytryptamine (5-HT), which is known to play an important role in migraine. Many types of receptor for 5-HT exist and drugs like **methysergide** (an antagonist at 5-HT$_2$ and 5-HT$_{1c}$ subtypes) and the indole sulphonamide **GR-43175** (an agonist at 5-HT$_1$-like receptors) both have antimigraine effects.

Many other α-adrenoceptor blockers have been developed. **Phentolamine** and **tolazoline** are both competitive but neither shows much selectivity between the α-receptor subtypes. **Phenoxybenzamine** causes an irreversible blockade by binding covalently to the α-receptors but its actions are complex since it also blocks receptors for histamine (H$_1$), acetylcholine (muscarinic) and 5-HT as well as blocking NA uptake (uptake$_1$). A drug with high selectivity for the α_1-adrenoceptor subtype is **prazosin**, which produces vasodilatation and is used to treat hypertension. TFFTT

MCQ 73

Drugs which competitively block β-adrenoceptors

1. will antagonize both the cardiac and the vasopressor actions of **adrenaline**.
2. can also exhibit intrinsic sympathomimetic activity as does **dichloro-isoprenaline**.
3. can only be used safely as antihypertensive agents if they are selective towards β_2-adrenoceptors.
4. may be used to treat the symptoms of hyperthyroidism.
5. should not be used in compensated congestive heart disease since they may precipitate cardiac failure.

There are differences between β-adrenoceptor blocking drugs with respect to:

(a) the degree of selectivity between β_1- and β_2-subtypes;
(b) the amount of partial agonist activity (sometimes called intrinsic sympathomimetic activity; ISA);
(c) possession of membrane-stabilizing activity (sometimes called local anaesthetic action or quinidine-like effect);
(d) lipid solubility, which governs the passage of the drug across cell membranes and hence the likelihood of CNS effects;
(e) potency in blocking β-adrenoceptors.

After the discovery (in the late 1950s) of β-adrenoceptor blocking actions in the partial agonist **dichloroisoprenaline**, a decade of research produced several useful drugs. **Propranolol** is the standard antagonist with which to compare new blockers. It is non-selective between β-adrenoceptor subtypes, has local anaesthetic activity with a potency similar to **procaine**, lacks ISA and is lipid-soluble. **Propranolol** was used first to treat angina and later against cardiac dysrhythmias, especially when catecholamines contribute to the condition. Its current major therapeutic outlet (as an antihypertensive) was discovered during early clinical use. **Propranolol** is very effective against the cardiotonic activity seen in hyperthyroidism (through cardiac β-adrenoceptor blockade and also through inhibiting the conversion of thyroxine to tri-iodothyronine in the plasma). Additionally, some types of tremor are reduced, migraine has been relieved and certain anxiety syndromes have been alleviated.

Clinically undesirable effects of **propranolol** are generally minor. Sedation, sleep disturbances and depression result from its access to the CNS. However, the major problems during drug therapy are predictable from the β-adrenoceptor blockade. Pre-existing asthma and other types of airway obstruction are likely to be worsened. Patients with myocardial infarction or compensated congestive heart disease are at risk since the cardiac depressant action of **propranolol** may provoke fatal heart failure. In such cases of cardiac or respiratory deficit the patient is dependent on endogenous catecholamines to minimize the severity of his condition. β-Adrenoceptor blockade will remove the support given to the cardiac and respiratory systems by the sympathetic nervous system and will thus exacerbate the condition. FTFTT

β-Blocking agents which are selective towards β₁-adrenoceptors

1. are relatively ineffective in antagonizing vasodilatation caused by **isoprenaline**.
2. include **practolol, atenolol** and **acebutolol**.
3. are useful in the treatment of asthma.
4. lack CNS activity because β-adrenoceptors are not found in the brain.
5. affect only cardiac function.

Once it was established that the β-adrenoceptors of the heart (β₁) were different from those of the bronchioles (β₂), it was appreciated that β-adrenoceptor blockers with a selectivity between these subgroups might have clinical advantages. The clinical benefits, mainly due to blockade of cardiac β₁-adrenoceptors, could be obtained without the danger of precipitating an asthmatic attack in susceptible individuals (which occurs by antagonism of the dilator action of circulating adrenaline on the bronchioles). With this end in view, **practolol**, a β₁-adrenoceptor blocker with partial agonist action (intrinsic sympathomimetic activity; ISA) but no membrane-stabilizing (local anaesthetic) effect was developed and used extensively. Reports of toxicity on the cornea (leading to blindness) and the intestine (mesenteric sclerosing fibrosis leading to peritonitis) led to the drug's withdrawal. The later development of **atenolol** (which lacks both ISA and local anaesthetic actions) and **acebutolol** (which has both) filled the gap.

The clinical advantage conferred by these actions is controversial. Doubt has even been cast on the concept that selectivity for β₁-adrenoceptors is an advantage in the asthmatic patient. In spite of the elegant theory, there is evidence that precipitation of asthmatic attacks may be unrelated to blockade of the bronchial β-adrenoceptors.

β-Blockers are among the most frequently prescribed drugs to treat hypertension but despite exhaustive investigations their mode of action is unclear. The reduction in force and rate of cardiac contraction, due to the blockade of the effects of the sympathetic nervous system, occurs within an hour of oral administration, while the antihypertensive effect takes several days to develop. The antihypertensive effect is not on the CNS since β-blockers with different abilities to penetrate the CNS (through differences in lipid solubility) all have similar antihypertensive actions. Production of renin (and ultimately angiotensin) is inhibited by β₂-adrenoceptor blockers but even 'selective' β₁-adrenoceptor blockers will lower high blood pressure. A recent suggestion is that, by blocking presynaptic β-receptors (normally stimulated by circulating adrenaline which facilitates release of noradrenaline), these drugs diminish the amount of noradrenaline liberated, leading to an antihypertensive effect. It will be interesting to see if this theory survives the test of time any better than its predecessors. TTFFF

MCQ 75

A pharmacological comparison of isolated atria and vas deferens shows that

1. ganglion blocking drugs reduce the effects of transmural electrical stimulation in both preparations.
2. ganglion blocking drugs reduce the effects of stimulating the attached vagal or hypogastric nerve fibres.
3. **botulinum toxin** will block the atrial tachycardia and the contraction of the vas deferens produced by transmural stimulation.
4. **prazosin** will reduce the response of the vas deferens but not that of the atria to transmural stimulation.
5. **isoprenaline** will cause atrial tachycardia and contraction of the vas deferens.

Isolated atria beat spontaneously because of sinoatrial nodal activity. Stimulation of parasympathetic (vagal, releasing acetylcholine; ACh) or sympathetic nerves (releasing noradrenaline; NA) produces a bradycardia or a tachycardia respectively, the size depending on the frequency of stimulation. The force of atrial contraction (measured isometrically) is also decreased (ACh) or increased (NA) by stimulating the appropriate nerves. If stimulation is transmural, the two effects are antagonistic and the result is unpredictable (unless the parasympathetic component is eliminated by the inclusion of **atropine** in the solution whereupon positive chronotropic and positive inotropic effects occur on stimulation).

If a drug blocks the effects of both vagal and preganglionic sympathetic stimulation, but does not reduce the actions of exogenous **NA** and **ACh**, it is likely to act by either ganglion blockade or local anaesthesia. A ganglion blocker would be ineffective against transmural stimulation, whereas a local anaesthetic would block this response too. In vas deferens, a ganglion blocker like **hexamethonium** would block the response to hypogastric nerve stimulation, but not the response to transmural stimulation.

A drug acting solely on neuronal processes will block the response to stimulation but not to added agonists. Examples are: local anaesthetics (like **lignocaine**), affecting all nerves; **botulinum toxin**, affecting only cholinergic nerves; and adrenergic neurone blockers (like **guanethidine**), affecting mainly noradrenergic nerves.

Striking differences in effect will be apparent between sympathomimetics which are selective towards presynaptic (mainly α_2) or postsynaptic adrenoceptors (in heart β_1 and in vas deferens mainly α_1). The α_2-adrenoceptor stimulant **clonidine** will activate the feedback mechanism which suppresses NA release and will reduce both the tachycardia and the contraction of the vas deferens produced by stimulation. **Phenylephrine** (α_1-adrenoceptor stimulant) has little effect on atria but will contract the vas deferens or summate with the sympathetic stimulation. **Prazosin** (an α_1-adrenoceptor blocker) will reduce the response of the vas deferens but have little effect on the response of the atria.

β-Blockers like **propranolol** reduce sympathomimetic actions of drugs on atria by postsynaptic blockade. β-Stimulants like **isoprenaline** produce tachycardia and will inhibit the response of the vas deferens to stimulation by activating relaxant β-adrenoceptors. FTFTF

In pharmacological investigations on isolated tissues

1. responses to field stimulation result from excitation of postganglionic nerves.
2. stimulation with an electrode placed on the vagal trunk excites preganglionic fibres.
3. a drug may affect the response to autonomic nerve stimulation by interacting with presynaptic purinoceptors.
4. a drug blocking stimulation by a presynaptic action will also block the response to exogenous transmitter.
5. only one transmitter is released in response to electrical stimulation of the intestine.

Many receptors exist postsynaptically (where their stimulation may modify the activity of the effector organ) and many exist presynaptically (where their stimulation may modify neurotransmitter release). The effects of agonists or antagonists at any of these sites can usually be examined in tissues that have been removed from the body along with their attached nerves, which can be stimulated through contact electrodes. In the case of the parasympathetic system any efferent nerve entering an organ will be entirely preganglionic, the ganglia themselves (with the exception of the ciliary ganglion) being embedded in the tissue close to the effector cells. In the sympathetic system the efferent nerves entering the tissue are generally postganglionic, the cell bodies themselves being located in the distant para- or prevertebral sympathetic ganglia. It is sometimes possible to obtain a sufficient length of sympathetic nerve for electrodes to be placed both pre- and postganglionically (e.g. in rabbit atria) and drug actions at either site examined.

An alternative method of applying electrical stimulation is to use a 'field' of current (transmural or coaxial stimulation). If current is passed between two parallel platinum wires, one on either side of a tissue mounted in a balanced physiological saline solution, both pre- and postganglionic fibres will be excited with a suitable current pulse. Postganglionic excitation will be propagated to the terminal varicosities and cause transmitter release, while preganglionic excitation will peter out as the propagated action potential finds the postganglionic nerve in its refractory period having also just been stimulated. The end-organ response, therefore, is due just to postganglionic stimulation.

It should be noted that *all* nerves, regardless of their origin or biochemical characteristics, will be excited by field stimulation. The response of the tissue could, therefore, be a combination of the effects of several transmitters. In gut muscle, noradrenaline, acetylcholine, dopamine, purines and polypeptides have all been postulated as transmitters. The effects of drugs could be brought about by supplementing or antagonizing the effects of any of these substances at pre- or postsynaptic sites. Generally these can be distinguished since presynaptic blockers usually have little effect on exogenous transmitter acting postsynaptically. TTTFF

Cardiovascular System

Disorders of cardiovascular function

1. include congestive heart failure, which may be treated with inotropic agents.
2. may be produced by **digitalis**.
3. include high blood pressure, which can be successfully treated with drugs in more than 90% of patients.
4. may result from increased plasma levels of some lipoproteins.
5. can usually be cured by aptly chosen drugs.

Understanding how drugs may affect the cardiovascular system is helped by knowing its physiology. The isolated heart will beat in a rhythmic, coordinated manner, but *in vivo* its rate and force are influenced by both sympathetic (increased) and parasympathetic (decreased) nervous systems. Vascular smooth muscle receives only a sympathetic innervation (noradrenaline causes vasoconstriction) but responds to a variety of blood-borne chemicals, many of which help to regulate vascular tone. Systemic blood pressure is the product of cardiac output (heart rate × stroke volume) and vascular resistance to blood flow (arterioles being the major vessels involved). Increased sympathetic activity would increase blood pressure through both cardiac and vascular changes. Increased parasympathetic activity would cause the blood pressure to fall by affecting the heart alone. It is vitally important that, over a range of blood pressure values, an adequate blood flow is maintained to organs like the brain, kidneys and the heart muscle itself. A variety of mechanisms exist for this purpose, some with widespread effects (e.g. baroreceptor reflexes, hormone release), others more restricted (e.g. metabolites, local hormones, autacoids).

There are many disorders of the cardiovascular system amenable to drug therapy; drugs alleviate but rarely cure the disorders. For instance, antidysrhythmic drugs may restore a regular heart beat; inotropic agents may promote a more forceful beat in patients with congestive heart failure; for patients with myocardial ischaemia (causing the chest pain, angina pectoris) there are substances which reduce cardiac work or which improve coronary blood flow; high blood pressure (which may lead to strokes and to damage of vulnerable organs) may be lowered to comparatively safe levels by a variety of drugs, given alone or in combination, providing successful treatment in over 90% of hypertensive patients.

Conversely, there are drugs used for a variety of other purposes which cause undesirable effects by additional actions on the cardiovascular system. In some cases the side-effects can be predicted from a knowledge of a drug's mechanism of action. For instance, **isoprenaline** relieves the bronchoconstriction of asthma by stimulating β_2-adrenoceptors in airways to relax the smooth muscle but it also stimulates cardiac β_1-adrenoceptors to increase rate and force of heart contraction; in high concentrations it may induce fatal cardiac dysrhythmias. Digitalis glycosides are used to treat congestive heart failure and certain atrial tachycardias, but may provoke many types of dysrhythmia, the most dangerous being ventricular fibrillation. In other cases cardiovascular side-effects may be less easily explained by a

continued on next page

drug's known mode of action (e.g. the orthostatic hypotension occurring early in therapy in about a third of the patients given **levodopa** for parkinsonism).

Some cardiovascular complaints arise because of disturbances or deficiencies in the composition of the blood. For instance, narrowing of arteries by atheromatous deposits is associated with high plasma levels of certain lipoproteins; individuals so affected are at increased risk of heart attacks and strokes. Drugs are known which reduce elevated levels of plasma lipids, though their success in reducing mortality from cardiovascular events is not proven. Other blood factors contributing to circulatory disorders are platelets and the proteins of the coagulation system. TTTTF

The vascular endothelium

1. releases both vasoconstrictor and vasodilator substances.
2. possesses muscarinic receptors which respond to acetylcholine.
3. liberates arachidonic acid metabolites such as thromboxane A_2.
4. must be intact for **nitroprusside** to produce its vasodilatation.
5. inactivates bradykinin and generates angiotensin II.

Vascular endothelium is important in the following ways:

(a) angiotensin converting enzyme, found on the outer surface of endothelial cells, biotransforms an inactive precursor to the vasoconstrictor peptide angiotensin II and inactivates the vasodilator peptide bradykinin;
(b) endothelial cells can take up and metabolize other vasoactive materials (e.g. 5-hydroxytryptamine (5-HT), adenosine);
(c) the cells can respond to a variety of chemical or physical stimuli to synthesize and release vasodilator substances such as the arachidonic acid metabolite prostacyclin (PGI_2) and the labile endothelium-derived relaxing factor (EDRF);
(d) the release of a vasoconstrictor peptide (endothelin) has been detected from cultured endothelial cells, although there is debate as to whether it, or yet another endothelial substance, is responsible for the vascular contractions generated by hypoxia.

The finding that in some vascular preparations acetylcholine (ACh) caused contraction but in others caused relaxation was resolved in 1980 by the discovery that an intact endothelium was required for the latter response. Damage to or removal of the endothelium prevented the relaxation caused by liberation of EDRF on stimulation of muscarinic receptors. Endothelium-derived relaxing factor, which is not stored but is synthesized on demand, can also be released by bradykinin, histamine and 5-HT among others. Like PGI_2, EDRF suppresses platelet aggregation and counteracts the vaso-constriction caused, for example by the arachidonic acid metabolite thromboxane A_2. The effects of EDRF are mediated by activation of guanylate cyclase, which results in elevation of cyclic-GMP levels. Activation of this enzyme also occurs with vasodilator drugs like **glyceryl trinitrate** and **nitroprusside**, but only after they have been biotransformed to nitric oxide (NO). The similarity in their effect led to comparative studies of EDRF and NO. Relaxation of isolated vascular muscle to NO and EDRF followed the same time course; both were inhibited by haemoglobin (which binds NO) and potentiated by the enzyme superoxide dismutase; their actions on platelets were identical and chemical assays showed that NO was liberated by cultured endothelial cells. Therefore it appears that EDRF is nitric oxide.

Thus the vascular endothelium plays an important role in the regulation of vascular tone, not only by contributing to the removal or activation of vasoactive substances but also by producing a range of materials itself. Some drugs may cause their vascular effects indirectly, by a primary action on the endothelial cells. TTFFT

MCQ 79

The renin–angiotensin system

1. is stimulated by increases in blood pressure or blood volume.
2. produces an octapeptide, angiotensin II, which causes aldosterone release.
3. may be attenuated by β-adrenoceptor blockers, which inhibit renin release.
4. is augmented when angiotensin-converting enzyme is blocked, since angiotensin II will be preserved.
5. may be involved in CNS neurotransmission.

The renin–angiotensin (R–A) system has important homeostatic functions and drugs affecting its activity are used therapeutically against hypertension and congestive heart failure. A protease (renin), released by the juxta-glomerular cells of the kidney, splits a decapeptide, angiotensin I, from a plasma globulin precursor. Renin release is stimulated by falls in blood volume or pressure, by Na^+ depletion or by increased sympathetic activity acting via β_1-adrenoceptors on the juxtaglomerular cells. Angiotensin I is converted to the active octapeptide angiotensin II by angiotensin-converting enzyme (ACE), found chiefly on the luminal surface of vascular endothelial cells. Angiotensin-converting enzyme also inactivates the vasodilator nonapeptide, bradykinin.

Angiotensin II causes vasoconstriction and also stimulates adrenal cortical cells to liberate aldosterone (a hormone acting on the kidney to cause Na^+ retention at the expense of K^+ and H^+). These effects counteract some of the stimuli for renin release. Since all the components of the R–A system have been found in the brain, angiotensin II is a putative transmitter or modulator and is thought to play a part in thirst and in regulation of sympathetic tone.

Because of its direct and indirect effects on the cardiovascular system, the R–A system has been implicated in hypertension, although high levels of plasma renin have not been uniformly found in patients with high blood pressure. However, drugs blocking the R–A system have been shown to lower blood pressure in many patients.

Saralasin, an octapeptide, is a partial agonist at vascular angiotensin receptors and was shown to lower the blood pressure in patients with hypertension associated with renal dysfunction. The need to give **saralasin** i.v. and the fact that some patients responded with increased blood pressure made it unsuitable for therapy. However, clinical success has been achieved with ACE inhibitors, substances which block the production but not the actions of angiotensin II. First **teprotide**, followed by the orally active **captopril** and, more recently, the pro-drug **enalapril** have been used in the treatment of high blood pressure. Their action is principally to cause a reduction in arteriolar resistance with little effect on heart rate or on baroreceptor function. Although the vascular effect can be explained by reduced synthesis of angiotensin II, there may be a contribution from the vasodilator peptide bradykinin, whose breakdown is concurrently prevented when ACE is blocked. Aldosterone release can still be maintained

continued on next page

via other stimuli such as corticotrophin (adrenocorticotrophic hormone) or K$^+$. Undesirable effects are few, though skin rashes have been reported with **captopril**, possibly a consequence of its sulphydryl groups, absent in **enalapril**, which has a lower tendency to cause rashes.

In future, drugs which inhibit renin may be developed for clinical trial. Such compounds might share many of the properties of ACE inhibitors since angiotensin II formation would be blocked at an earlier stage, though bradykinin metabolism would be unaffected. It should be noted that β-adrenoceptor blocking agents are able to reduce renin release by their action on juxtaglomerular cells, an effect which may contribute to their antihypertensive activity in some patients. FTTFT

MCQ 80

Drugs generally referred to as 'calcium channel blockers'

1. prevent the escape of Ca^{2+} from cells.
2. include **prenylamine** and **verapamil**.
3. relax arterial smooth muscle.
4. may be used to treat atrial dysrhythmias (e.g. **diltiazem**).
5. include **nifedipine**, which has antianginal and antihypertensive activity.

Increase in concentration of free Ca^{2+} within cells usually activates them (e.g. gland cells to secrete, muscle cells to contract). Elevation of $[Ca^{2+}]$ can occur by release of ions from intracellular storage sites like mitochondrial or reticular membranes or by influx of Ca^{2+} from extracellular fluid. Basically two types of membrane channels exist through which Ca^{2+} enters cells:

(a) receptor-operated (ROC), about which little is known currently and for which no selective blockers exist;
(b) voltage-operated (VOC), which open when cell membranes are depolarized by stimuli such as K^+.

Several classes of chemicals are known which block VOC (e.g. dihydropyridines, phenylalkylamines, benzothiazepines) and some workers suggest that each class is site-specific. A dihydropyridine (**BAY K8644**) has been discovered which opens Ca^{2+} channels. Moreover, the *state* of VOC (whether resting, open or inactivated) may affect the binding of these drugs, so their actions are unlikely to be uniform in all tissues despite the wide distribution of VOC.

In the heart, depolarization of conducting tissue and muscle cells is brought about by inward movement of Na^+ (fast channel) and then Ca^{2+} (slow). After opening to allow Ca^{2+} entry, channels undergo a recovery period before they conduct more ions. Drugs affecting channel function may simply reduce Ca^{2+} entry whilst the channels are open or may lengthen the recovery time. **Nifedipine** (a dihydropyridine) does not slow recovery and has relatively less effect on the heart than drugs like **prenylamine**, **verapamil** and **diltiazem**, which do. Thus these last drugs are employed clinically in the treatment of cardiac dysrhythmias (especially atrial, which involve a higher discharge frequency) and are classified as Type IV antidysrhythmic drugs.

Depolarization of vascular smooth muscle is dependent on Ca^{2+} entry (not Na^+) and calcium channel blockers effectively cause relaxation. Arteriolar muscle is more sensitive than venular; and dihydropyridines tend to be more effective than the other classes on vascular preparations. Thus **nifedipine** is used in the treatment of angina pectoris. By its peripheral vasodilating actions it reduces the workload on the heart and it also improves perfusion of the myocardial vascular bed. It depresses myocardial contractility less than the other drugs for the reasons given above. **Diltiazem** is also used in angina.

Dihydropyridines in particular are receiving attention as antihypertensive agents and **nifedipine** is being used increasingly, either alone or, more

 continued on next page

usually, in combination with other drugs. As more Ca^{2+} entry blockers are discovered, they are likely to offer a wider choice to clinicians not only in the therapy of hypertension, but in other areas too. For example, in future, such drugs might be used in the treatment of asthma (by relaxation of bronchial smooth muscle); of biliary colic and localized spasm of other areas of the gastrointestinal tract; and, because of actions in depressing neuronal activity, they might find applications in analgesia or against convulsive disorders. FTTTT

Hypertension

1. is a sustained muscular contraction associated with anxiety.
2. if prolonged, leads to vascular damage especially in the eye and brain.
3. is unaffected by psychotherapy.
4. is classified as essential when the cause is unknown.
5. is diagnosed when the systolic blood pressure reaches 90 mmHg

Some estimates suggest that between 10 and 20% of adults in Western societies have a sufficiently high arterial blood pressure to warrant medical treatment. Prolonged hypertension damages blood vessels in the eye, kidney, brain and heart, resulting in retinopathy, renal failure, stroke and coronary disease respectively. Hypertension is often associated with atherosclerosis (vascular narrowing through deposition of lipoproteins (plaque) in the arterial wall) and there is an increased incidence of thromboembolic (blood clotting) disorders. The expectation of life is reduced by an extent related to the degree of hypertension.

An increase in diastolic blood pressure (normally 70–80 mmHg) is clinically more significant than a rise in systolic blood pressure (normally 120–140 mmHg). Diastolic pressure normally rises with age but mild hypertension would probably be diagnosed at values over 90 mmHg, moderate at about 120 mmHg and severe at over 150 mmHg. In only 10% of cases is the cause of the hypertension known (e.g. renal insufficiency, phaeochromocytoma) and in the remainder the condition is called 'essential hypertension'. Several factors predispose to hypertension including a family history of the condition, diet (especially salt intake), smoking and psychological stress. Removal of these predisposing factors is among the most beneficial methods of preventing and treating hypertension, the most successful being weight loss in the obese hypertensive individual and restriction of salt intake. Indeed, a reduction in salt intake to about 80 mEq daily can be as effective as treatment with, for example, diuretic drugs, although only about half the hypertensive population is likely to respond.

Blood pressure is proportional to cardiac output (dependent on heart rate and stroke volume) and total peripheral resistance (dependent on the degree of vasoconstriction). Neuronal and hormonal mechanisms adjust the blood pressure and appear to be 'set' at a higher than normal level in hypertension. Drug treatment of essential hypertension is usually directed at the sign (i.e the high blood pressure) since the cause is generally unknown, so it is important to balance the potential benefit against the possible harm caused by antihypertensive drugs, which will probably have to be given for life.

The decision when to start drug therapy in a patient with mild hypertension is a difficult one. There are many drugs available to treat essential hypertension which may be used alone or in combination but none cures the disease and all are associated with some unwanted effects. FTFTF

The pharmacological management of hypertension

1. can be achieved in over 90% of patients at low therapeutic cost.
2. usually begins when the cause of the hypertension has been identified.
3. is likely to start with the prescription of a diuretic drug along with a sodium dietary supplement.
4. is unlikely nowadays to involve vasodilator drugs.
5. may involve concurrent administration of as many as three different types of drug.

Sustained hypertension can be lowered by several different mechanisms. Since blood pressure is proportional to cardiac output and total peripheral resistance, drugs could theoretically work by reducing heart rate and/or stroke volume and/or peripheral resistance, although a reduction in any one of these frequently brings about a reflex compensatory rise in the others. In addition, reductions in the volume of circulating fluid (e.g. by increasing the excretion of Na^+, and therefore water, by the kidney) will also reduce blood pressure. Frequently hypertension is better controlled by low doses of several drugs acting by different mechanisms rather than by a high dose of a single agent and, towards this end, a stepped approach is used in clinical management.

Commonly, treatment of mild or moderate hypertension begins with increasing doses of a single drug until the desired effect or a maximum tolerated dose has been reached. In stage 1, a diuretic drug (e.g. a thiazide such as **chlorothiazide**) or a β-adrenoceptor blocking agent would normally be given. If this proved inadequate then, in stage 2, a combination of the two types of drug would be tried. If the combination caused toxic effects or failed to control the high blood pressure, then inhibitors of the renin–angiotensin system (e.g. **captopril, enalapril**) might be substituted. Alternatively in stage 2 the diuretic could be accompanied by a different sort of drug affecting sympathetic function, since diminished sympathetic activity leads to a reduction in vasoconstriction and hence lowers peripheral resistance. Drugs may cause this effect by acting primarily on the CNS (**clonidine, α-methyldopa**). Some agents may affect multiple sites or act by mechanisms which are not fully understood (e.g. β-adrenoceptor blockers). **Prazosin** blocks α_1-adrenoceptors and may have CNS actions in addition to directly producing vascular relaxation.

If any combination of two drugs fails to work, then stage 3 requires the addition of a third substance. There is no point in using drugs from the same pharmacological class, so the next would be aptly chosen from a list including **captopril** (an inhibitor of angiotensin-converting enzyme) or vasodilator substances (e.g. **hydrallazine, minoxidil**) acting on the blood vessels to reduce peripheral resistance. Their mechanisms vary, but **nitroprusside** acts by being metabolized to nitric oxide, while others (e.g. **nifedipine**) reduce the availability of intracellular calcium ions.

In extreme cases a fourth drug (e.g. **guanethidine**, an adrenergic neurone blocker) may be added to the combination. With the stepped approach to therapy, an adequate control of blood pressure can be achieved in more than 90% of patients.

continued on next page 103

The term therapeutic cost does not describe the monetary cost of the treatment given. All drug treatments cause some discomfort or risk of harm to the patient and it is this which is referred to as the therapeutic cost. This is especially important in conditions like hypertension, where drug treatment may continue for many years. TFFFT

Diuretics

1. are drugs with a primary action on the glomerulus of the kidney.
2. may be used in the treatment of diabetes insipidus because they can reduce water loss from the kidney.
3. are used to reduce plasma potassium levels and thereby lower **digitalis** toxicity in patients with congestive heart failure.
4. may act on the collecting tubules by antagonizing aldosterone.
5. include the sulphonamide drugs **frusemide** and **hydrochlorothiazide**.

Diuretic drugs are used to treat a variety of conditions where electrolyte imbalance occurs but their principal use is in the treatment of hypertension. They can act by several mechanisms.

Thiazides (e.g. **chlorothiazide**, **hydrochlorothiazide**) increase the urinary output of Na^+ by decreasing the reabsorption of NaCl in the first segment of the distal tubule, though little is known about the transport mechanism which is inhibited. Paradoxically, thiazides produce an *anti*diuretic effect in patients with diabetes insipidus and this may be due to the ability of thiazides to increase tubular permeability to water, a property most evident in circumstances where tubular permeability is at its lowest. Many thiazides are available. They all possess an unsubstituted sulphonamide group which is essential for their diuretic activity but lack the *p*-amino group which is necessary for antibacterial activity. Like many other types of diuretic drug, thiazides cause hypokalaemia by promoting K^+ loss. It may be necessary to give dietary K^+ supplements to patients receiving these drugs, and especially if the patients are concurrently receiving **digitalis** for congestive heart failure. **Digitalis glycosides** have a low therapeutic index and are especially toxic during hypokalaemic states (possibly because of the increased vulnerability of the ATPase which the glycosides block).

Another class of diuretic drugs acts on the loop of Henle, which has a large absorptive capacity for Na^+. Drugs such as **frusemide** (another sulphonamide), its analogues **bumetanide** and **piretanide**, as well as the chemically unrelated **ethacrynic acid**, act here and cause considerable diuresis. The diuresis is too large for their *routine* use as antihypertensive drugs but they are used in severe hypertension, pulmonary oedema and hypercalcaemia. Predictably, they cause considerable K^+ loss and also H^+ loss, resulting in a hypokalaemic metabolic alkalosis. Care must be taken with these sulphonamide drugs since allergy is not uncommon and there may be cross-reactivity in patients sensitive to antibacterial sulphonamides.

Potassium-sparing diuretics exist, all working directly or indirectly on the cortical collecting tubules, where aldosterone normally acts to promote K^+ secretion into the lumen. These drugs work by

(a) antagonism at the aldosterone receptor (e.g. **spironolactone**);
(b) suppressing angiotensin II generation (e.g. **captopril**);
(c) directly inhibiting Na^+ transport in the collecting tubule (e.g. **triamterene**, **amiloride**).

Sometimes used in hypertension, they are also used in hyperaldosteronism.
FTFTT

MCQ 84

In the pharmacological management of hypertension

1. β-adrenoceptor blocking agents cause vasodilatation by acting on vascular β-adrenoceptors.
2. **propranolol** may give rise to rebound tachycardia and nervousness when therapy is stopped.
3. selective β_1-adrenoceptor blockers are of little use as they affect only the heart.
4. **clonidine** is used as it lacks central side-effects.
5. **clonidine** acts by blockade of presynaptic α_2-adrenoceptors, thereby reducing noradrenaline release.

The most commonly used antihypertensive agents which interfere with sympathetic function are the β-adrenoceptor blocking agents ('β-blockers', e.g. **propranolol**). The precise mechanism by which they lower blood pressure is unclear although β_1-adrenoceptors appear to be involved, since selective blockers of this subtype (e.g. **atenolol, metoprolol**) are antihypertensive. All these drugs block cardiac β-adrenoceptors but, while this action can be demonstrated within hours of administration, the antihypertensive effect takes several days to occur. Renin release from the kidney is inhibited and therefore a contribution to the antihypertensive effect may come from the subsequent reduction in levels of the vasoconstrictor peptide angiotensin II. A CNS action has been postulated, but some effective β-blockers (e.g. **atenolol**) penetrate the CNS poorly. The lowered blood pressure cannot be explained by an action on vascular β-adrenoceptors, since these belong to the β_2-subtype and mediate vasodilatation when *agonists* bind to them. Certain undesirable effects, however, are predictable from β-adrenoceptor blockade, for example bronchoconstriction, hypoglycaemia and negative chronotropic and inotropic effects; and, from those penetrating the CNS, sedation, sleep disturbances and depression. An 'abstinence syndrome' has been reported on abrupt cessation of therapy which includes nervousness, tachycardia and angina.

Less frequently used nowadays because of a spectrum of undesirable effects is **clonidine**, an imidazoline which acts on the CNS. It decreases the discharge from the vasomotor centre, causing a reduction in arteriolar resistance and a fall in blood pressure. **Clonidine** has been shown to stimulate α-adrenoceptors on neurones in the medulla (and hypothalamus), which leads to a reduction in the firing rate of efferent sympathetic nerves; in the periphery, α_2-adrenoceptors are autoinhibitory and therefore **clonidine** can reduce the output of noradrenaline from stimulated nerves. Its weak agonist actions on α_1-adrenoceptors may result in an initial pressor response if given i.v.

Clonidine causes a dry mouth and sedation (both CNS effects). It may aggravate or even precipitate depression and should be withdrawn from patients suffering depression. On withdrawal many patients suffer 'rebound hypertension'. Tachycardia, nervousness, headache and sweating are common and may occur if one or two doses of the drug are missed during therapy. Although its clinical use has declined, **clonidine** remains an important tool in pharmacological research. FTFFF

In the therapy of hypertension

1. diuretic agents should not be used for longer than 2 months since by this time blood volume has returned to original levels.
2. a combination of a diuretic and a β-adrenoceptor blocking drug causes postural hypotension.
3. vasodilator drugs like **hydrallazine** are usually given alone.
4. **prazosin** causes less tachycardia than other α-adrenoceptor blocking drugs because it selectively blocks α-adrenoceptors.
5. a combination of drugs like **chlorothiazide**, **propranolol** and **prazosin** could commonly be employed.

Reduced dietary sodium intake may produce a modest antihypertensive effect in many people, so it is not surprising that diuretics have a primary role in the treatment of hypertension. Initially these drugs lower blood pressure by reducing blood volume and cardiac output and may cause a reflex increase in total peripheral resistance during the first few weeks of treatment. Usually, by 2 months, cardiac output has returned to normal but blood pressure remains lower and total peripheral resistance is also reduced at this time, possibly due to a change in vessel stiffness which is sensitive to Na^+. Sometimes a potassium-sparing diuretic (e.g. **spironolactone**) may be given in combination with a thiazide and the combination will produce less disturbance in K^+ levels, which may be critical (e.g. in patients taking **digitalis**).

In 30–40% of patients a diuretic drug alone will not provide adequate control of the hypertension and it is then usual to substitute a β-blocker (e.g. **propranolol**) or to give the two agents together. The mode of action of β-adrenoceptor blocking drugs in lowering blood pressure is unclear but patients benefit from combined therapy because

(a) diuretics prevent the salt and water retention sometimes seen with β-blockers alone;
(b) diuretics stimulate the renin–angiotensin system, which tends to limit their antihypertensive action, but β-blockers suppress renin release;
(c) postural hypotension is uncommon with this combination.

In patients whose hypertension is inadequately controlled by this drug combination or in whom toxic effects are seen, either a third drug may be added or another drug substituted. Substances with direct or indirect vasodilatory actions are generally used at this stage.

Captopril blocks angiotensin-converting enzyme (ACE), thereby preventing the intravascular formation of the vasoconstrictor peptide angiotensin II. Inhibitors of ACE are increasingly used in earlier stages of therapy because of their effectiveness and relative lack of side-effects. **Nifedipine** blocks Ca^{2+} entry, especially into arteriolar smooth muscle, and so causes vasodilatation. **Prazosin** relaxes smooth muscle both in resistance and capacitance vessels by blocking postsynaptic α_1-adrenoceptors. It may additionally affect sympathetic outflow by an action on the CNS, which may contribute to the virtual absence of reflex tachycardia. The lack of

continued on next page 107

presynaptic α_2-adrenoceptor blockade by **prazosin** may also play a part in minimizing reflex tachycardia, since an intact autoinhibitory mechanism helps suppress the output of noradrenaline. By contrast with **prazosin**, the vasodilator drug **hydrallazine** acts solely on resistance vessels. Reflex tachycardia does occur and **hydrallazine** is usually prescribed together with a β-adrenoceptor blocker to attenuate the reflex. FFFFT

Of the antihypertensive drugs that work by interfering with sympathetic nervous system function

1. the most commonly used are adrenergic neurone blocking agents like **guanethidine**.
2. both ganglion blockers and adrenergic neurone blockers cause postural hypotension.
3. **α-methyldopa** works by competing with noradrenaline for vascular α-adrenoceptors.
4. **α-methyldopa** may cause lactation in men.
5. most cause increased libido by reducing sympathetic control of the urogenital tract.

Considerable changes have occurred since 1950 in the drug treatment of hypertension, many remedies now being virtually obsolete. For instance, ganglion blocking agents (e.g. **pempidine**, **mecamylamine**) and adrenergic neurone blocking agents (e.g. **guanethidine**) are hardly ever used. They all reduced, by different mechanisms, the release of noradrenaline (NA) from sympathetic postganglionic fibres. While this led to the withdrawal of vasoconstrictor tone and reduced blood pressure, many undesirable effects (e.g. postural hypotension, impotence) were also caused by inhibition of NA release.

During the 1960s and early 1970s **α-methyldopa** became one of the most commonly used antihypertensives. It had been shown *in vitro* to inhibit dopa decarboxylase but acts as a substrate for this enzyme, eventually (*in vivo*) being converted into α-methylnoradrenaline. This 'false transmitter' replaces NA in the storage vesicles and is released from sympathetic nerves. However, α-methylnoradrenaline is only slightly less potent than NA at vascular α-adrenoceptors and this false transmitter function could not explain fully the antihypertensive effect, which is now known to be centrally, not peripherally, mediated. **α-Methyldopa** given intracerebroventricularly will reduce the blood pressure at much lower doses than when given i.v. Moreover, when inhibitors of dopa decarboxylase are given *centrally*, the antihypertensive action of **α-methyldopa** is blocked, while this does not occur when *peripheral* dopa decarboxylase is inhibited. It must, therefore, be converted to α-methylnoradrenaline which acts within the CNS.

α-Methyldopa (1–2 g daily) is effective in moderate hypertension and causes little postural hypotension. It frequently produces marked sedation and impairs mental concentration. Extrapyramidal effects occur occasionally as does lactation in both men and women, probably by an action on the hypothalamus. More serious are cases of autoimmune haemolytic anaemia. The development of antihypertensive therapies which are both effective and relatively free from associated unwanted effects has greatly reduced the popularity of **α-methyldopa**. FTFTF

MCQ 87

Myocardial ischaemia

1. is an alternative name for chest pain (angina pectoris).
2. may arise from coronary vasospasm.
3. is usually treated with drugs which selectively dilate the coronary vessels.
4. may be relieved by decreasing the workload on the heart.
5. occurs when cardiac oxygen demand exceeds supply.

Angina pectoris is the chest pain which is experienced when coronary blood cannot supply the heart muscle with sufficient oxygen, the deprived muscle being described as 'ischaemic'. Myocardial ischaemia, a common and serious health problem in the West, is usually caused by atheroma of coronary vessels but sometimes by spasm of the coronary vessels which transiently reduces the blood supply to parts of the heart. Classically, angina occurs when oxygen demand increases (e.g. during exercise), but the 'variant' angina which results from coronary spasm is caused by a reduction in oxygen delivery.

The oxygen consumption of the heart is high even under conditions of little stress, when about 75% of available oxygen is extracted from the blood to generate high-energy phosphates which supply the energy for cardiac work. Oxygen demand increases if there is a rise in heart rate, contractility, ventricular volume or blood pressure, for instance in exercise or even in preparing mentally for exercise. The demand for more oxygen can only be met by increasing coronary flow since oxygen carriage and extraction are almost maximal even at rest. Thus, in a patient with an obstruction to coronary flow, ischaemia and then angina could readily occur.

Whatever the type of angina, treatment attempts to improve coronary blood flow and/or reduce myocardial oxygen demand. Pharmacologically this is achieved with two different types of drug. One type dilates blood vessels and used to be termed 'coronary vasodilator' (organic nitrates and nitrites, and calcium influx inhibitors). It is now realized that such drugs act principally by dilating peripheral blood vessels, reducing blood pressure and, therefore, decreasing cardiac work and hence oxygen demand. The other type of drug is the β-adrenoceptor blocker, which prevents the heart from responding to sympathetic drive and therefore maintains heart work and oxygen demand at a low level even during exercise.

In classical angina caused by effort, drugs may provide effective treatment, but in the case of permanently narrowed or partially obstructed vessels only surgery can fully restore coronary blood supply. In variant angina, where the obstruction is due to vasospasm, drugs can also be effective.

If a major coronary vessel suddenly becomes occluded (more likely in vessels narrowed by atheromatous deposits), then the heart muscle supplied by it loses its nutrient and oxygen supply, which may lead to death of the muscle and prove fatal to the patient. A cardiac infarction has occurred and is signalled by the intense pain, shock and collapse that constitute a heart attack. Such a grave event should not be confused with angina pectoris, which signals ischaemia rather than infarction. FTFTT

In the management of angina pectoris

1. β-adrenoceptor blocking drugs are preferred for 'variant' angina (caused by coronary vasospasm).
2. vasodilator drugs like the organic nitrates are contraindicated in patients already receiving a β-blocker.
3. **verapamil** given together with a β-adrenoceptor blocking drug is contraindicated in patients also presenting with congestive heart failure.
4. **nifedipine** is useful in patients with low blood pressure because of its hypertensive effects.
5. 'calcium antagonists' increase tone of coronary arterial muscle.

β-Adrenoceptor blocking drugs (like **propranolol**) and 'calcium antagonists' are widely used in the management of angina. Regardless of the degree of selectivity for $β_1$- or $β_2$-adrenoceptors, there seems to be little difference between the β-blockers in effectiveness or in undesirable cardiac effects. The beneficial effects stem from the decreased heart rate, decreased contractility and, in hypertensive patients, the fall in blood pressure. This reduces the 'after-load' on the heart (i.e. the pressure against which the heart is working at the end of diastole). Exercise-induced (or 'classical') angina is especially responsive to β-blocking therapy as is the labile form ('unstable' angina), where attacks often occur in resting patients. Nitrates are sometimes given in combination with β-blocking drugs. This combination is useful because the β-blockers can reduce the reflex tachycardia which nitrates are liable to produce and because the increase in end-diastolic volume caused by β-blockers is counteracted by the reduction in end-diastolic volume caused by the nitrates.

Calcium antagonists are becoming more widely used especially for the treatment of 'variant angina', which appears to be caused by spasm of coronary arteries, thereby reducing blood flow. It has been estimated that these drugs can totally abolish variant angina attacks in more than two-thirds of patients and can produce some benefit in more than 90% of patients, presumably by preventing vasospasm. In stable chronic angina the benefits are thought to come from the decreased heart rate and contractility, which will reduce myocardial oxygen demand. **Nifedipine** produces a more pronounced hypotensive effect than **diltiazem** or **verapamil** and its relatively smaller direct effect on cardiac muscle means that sometimes a reflex tachycardia supervenes. The drugs may be used in combination with β-blockers, especially in the treatment of chronic angina, but caution is necessary. **Verapamil** and **diltiazem** combined with a β-blocker might eventually depress ventricular contractility and will usually worsen existing cardiac failure. **Nifedipine** should be avoided in patients with low blood pressure because of its hypotensive effects. Care must be taken in patients treated with **digitalis** because **verapamil** and **nifedipine** have been reported to increase **digoxin** plasma levels and the cardiac glycosides have a notoriously low therapeutic index. FFTFF

MCQ 89

Vasodilator drugs commonly used in the management of angina pectoris

1. include the explosive liquid **glyceryl trinitrate**.
2. may be administered through the skin or in sublingual tablets.
3. are beneficial because they dilate all the blood vessels of the body.
4. are the nitrates and nitrites, which may have a duration of action up to 6 h.
5. may give rise to intense headaches because they dilate meningeal vessels.

The vasodilators used in the treatment of angina are subdivided into the organic nitrates (and nitrites) and calcium entry blocking drugs. The former range from volatile liquids (**amyl nitrite**) to solids (**isosorbide dinitrate**). The explosive liquid **glyceryl trinitrate (nitroglycerin)** is prepared in a tablet form, small quantities being absorbed by inert fillers, therefore presenting no explosive hazard. The drug can be absorbed quickly from under the tongue (which reduces first pass biotransformation in the liver) or from ointments and impregnated plasters. **Amyl nitrite** is inhaled from a capsule crushed between the fingers.

Most of this group are short-acting drugs that are only active after transformation to the nitrite ion, which is thought to react with a specific receptor. Indeed, an endogenous vasodilator substance (endothelium-derived relaxing factor; EDRF), released from endothelial cells by a variety of stimuli, is now believed to be nitric oxide, which acts through the same receptor. Stimulation of the receptor activates guanylate cyclase, which causes elevation of intracellular cyclic-GMP levels, leading to muscle relaxation. The nitrates and nitrites cause all segments of the vascular system, arteries and veins, to relax and the eventual decrease in central venous pressure ('pre-load') helps reduce the work of the heart. Both angina and congestive heart failure are therefore relieved. Although reflexes bring about increased chronotropic and inotropic activity in response to the fall in blood pressure, the energy expenditure of the heart is still less than formerly.

Nitrites often cause a throbbing headache due to the dilatation of meningeal vessels and there is increased misuse of these drugs by teenagers and homosexual males because of the enhanced sexual excitement they cause. Tolerance readily occurs to the vasodilating properties. The nitrite ion can react with haemoglobin to form methaemoglobin, which has a lower affinity for oxygen. This is a potential hazard, especially when the intake of nitrates is high (overdose or from cured meats). The ability of these drugs to produce methaemoglobin is used in the treatment of cyanide poisoning since **cyanide** reacts preferentially with methaemoglobin and thus spares the essential cytochrome respiratory enzyme systems. Generally, because their action is short, the nitrites are used to treat attacks of angina rather than to prevent them (prophylactically). However, slowly absorbable preparations of **glyceryl trinitrate** produce proportionally higher plasma concentrations for longer periods and some orally administered drugs may act for up to 6 h. TTTTT

Cardiac dysrhythmias

1. may occur when drugs alter the rate of spontaneous depolarization in cardiac pacemaker cells.
2. may arise from a conduction disorder that causes the heart muscle to be excited more than once from a single impulse.
3. are likely to occur when normally quiescent cells assume a pacemaker function.
4. are made worse by high extracellular potassium levels.
5. due to 're-entry' of impulses may be treated either with drugs that shorten or with drugs that lengthen the refractory period of conducting tissue.

Cardiac dysrhythmias arise through disturbances in the initiation and/or conduction of electrical activity in the heart. They can at best provoke anxiety in patients and at worst lead to death from ventricular fibrillation. Many dysrhythmias are iatrogenic ('physician-induced'), caused by drugs prescribed for other purposes. About 25% of patients receiving cardiac glycosides will show dysrhythmias at some stage as will about 50% of patients anaesthetized for surgery. About 80% of patients with acute myocardial infarction will become dysrhythmic.

Pacemaker cells exist in various parts of the heart but are concentrated in the sinoatrial (SA) and atrioventricular (AV) nodes. These cells, unlike most others, slowly depolarize at rest until a critical potential is reached when a 'spike' potential arises and the electrical change is propagated through adjacent tissue. Many types of stimuli (chemical, mechanical, electrical) can alter the rate of this slow, spontaneous depolarization and hence change the frequency of spike discharge. Moreover, some normally quiescent (atrial or ventricular) cells can develop pacemaker activity in special circumstances, when potassium levels are low for example, or in the presence of various drugs.

Some dysrhythmias are caused when impulse conduction is severely depressed, leading to conditions like AV nodal block. A different conduction abnormality, called 're-entry', involves one impulse exciting the heart more than once. For re-entry to occur there must be: first, an obstacle to normal impulse flow; second, impulse conduction in one direction only in one branch of the bundle of His (i.e. unidirectional block); and third, a conduction time long enough for the re-entered tissue to be no longer refractory. The degree by which conduction is depressed in order for re-entry to occur is critical. The mechanism by which this occurs is in doubt but involves a decrease in the transmembrane flux of sodium or calcium or both.

Drugs may affect re-entry by improving or further depressing the critically depressed conduction in the region of a unidirectional block. This could occur by shortening or by lengthening the refractory period of the adjacent tissue. The shorter the refractory period, the less likely is unidirectional block, whilst the longer the period, the more likely is the tissue to be refractory when the re-entrant impulse arrives. Both actions would be antidysrhythmic. TTTFT

MCQ 91

Antidysrhythmic drugs may be classified on the basis of their mechanism of action,

1. **quinidine**, **phenytoin** and **lignocaine** being Class I because they all block sodium channels.
2. one group comprising drugs that oppose cardiac sympathetic activity.
3. **amiodarone** being Class III and lengthening the duration of the action potential by a mechanism other than sodium channel blockade.
4. the calcium antagonists (Class IV) like **verapamil** being used especially for disorders originating in the sinoatrial and atrioventricular nodes.
5. each class being used against a particular type of dysrhythmia.

It is the mechanism by which the antidysrhythmic drugs act which determines their class and some dysrhythmias may be remedied by drugs from several different classes.

Class I drugs act like local anaesthetics, blocking sodium channels and reducing the rate of rise of the action potential and the rate of spontaneous depolarization of pacemaker cells. The prototype is **quinidine**, others being **lignocaine**, **procainamide** and **phenytoin** (**diphenylhydantoin**). All their properties and uses derive from their ability to produce membrane stabilization by blocking sodium channels.

Class II agents act by opposing sympathetic activity on the heart. Typically, β-adrenoceptor blockers (**propranolol**, **atenolol**) fall into this group but it should be noted that some (e.g. **propranolol**) also have membrane-stabilizing activity, which may play some part in their action. These drugs are invaluable in treating dysrhythmias caused by sympathetic overactivity, such as might occur in hyperthyroidism, or when halogenated hydrocarbons, such as **halothane**, are used as general anaesthetics.

Class III drugs prolong the effective refractory period by lengthening the action potential through mechanisms other than acting on sodium channels. Only two drugs which are in clinical use fall into this category, **bretylium** and **amiodarone**. The former is recommended only for life-threatening ventricular dysrythmias which fail to respond to other treatments, and would be used i.v. in intensive care. **Amiodarone** is orally active, but plagued with a high incidence of adverse effects (including lung and liver lesions and peripheral neuropathy). Some unexpected deaths have occurred. A variety of mechanisms may contribute to its antidysrhythmic action, including slowing of K^+ efflux during repolarization and non-competitive blockade of α-and β-adrenoceptors.

Calcium is necessary for the maintenance of contractility in muscle and for normal conduction in specialized tissues in the heart. Voltage changes initiate the opening of Ca^{2+} channels (slow channels) which may be affected by drugs that simply reduce Ca^{2+} entry and/or slow the recovery of the activated channel. **Verapamil** has this latter effect and so is more active on tissues which fire frequently and which are less polarized at rest. It is therefore used especially to treat supraventricular dysrhythmias, i.e. those originating in the sinoatrial and atrioventricular nodes (the benefits arising from slowing the rate and lengthening the refractory period respectively). The Ca^{2+} entry blockers are known as *Class IV* drugs. Dihydropyridines (e.g. **nifedipine**) are more appropriately used against angina, because they principally cause vasodilatation, thereby helping reduce the workload on the heart. TTTTF

In the management of cardiac dysrhythmias

1. drug treatment may be withheld unless the disturbance is life-threatening.
2. reduction in the consumption of cigarettes, alcohol and coffee may be primary remedies.
3. **quinidine** is the drug of first choice for dysrhythmias due to myocardial infarction.
4. **lignocaine** is not given intravenously since it would rapidly penetrate the CNS.
5. **quinidine** has atropinic actions which counteract its action to depress pacemaker activity.

It is difficult to decide when to start treatment of dysrhythmias if the disorder does not threaten life. Atrial fibrillation carries a low risk of serious consequences and, since drug therapy is often unsuccessful, medication may be withheld. Counselling about risk factors is important, and patients should be advised against heavy exercise, psychological stress and certain foods as well as excessive smoking, **alcohol** and coffee consumption.

Many antidysrhythmic drugs depress left ventricular function (e.g. β-adrenoceptor blockers like **propranolol**) so care must be taken when they are used to treat atrioventricular nodal disturbances. In patients whose dysrhythmias are wholly ventricular the sodium channel blocking drugs (Class I; **quinidine, procainamide**) should also be used with great caution because they all depress left ventricular contractility. When dysrhythmias fail to respond to a given drug, combinations may be used, though usually not of drugs from the same class. Surgery or artificial pacemakers may have to be used if all attempts at drug therapy are unsuccessful.

Quinidine is one of the most common orally effective antidysrhythmic agents. It has many pharmacological effects including weak blocking actions at muscarinic and α-adrenoceptors, and antimalarial and antipyretic activity. It is effective in nearly every sort of dysrhythmia from atrial tachycardias through to ventricular extrasystoles. This wide spectrum of activity stems from the ability of **quinidine** to depress pacemaker rate and to decrease both excitability and conduction (particularly effectively in depolarized tissue). It also lengthens action potential duration. Its atropinic actions oppose the direct effect on sinoatrial nodal cells so that an actual increase in rate may occur in man where vagal tone is high (though not in the rat, where the main controlling influence on the resting heart is sympathetic). The most common undesirable effects are gastrointestinal upset and 'cinchonism' (dizziness, headache).

Procainamide is very similar in its actions to **quinidine** but has a short half-life, must be given very frequently and is less popular. **Lignocaine** (also Class I) is not effective orally because of extensive biotransformation in the liver and is usually given i.v. It is the drug of first choice in coronary care units to suppress ventricular tachycardias and to prevent fibrillation after myocardial infarction. It has few undesirable effects, although convulsions may occur in the elderly. TTFFT

MCQ 93

Among the drugs used to treat cardiac dysrhythmias

1. are the cardiac glycosides such as **digoxin**.
2. the β-adrenoceptor blocking agents appear to reduce the incidence of sudden death in patients recovering from myocardial infarction.
3. **verapamil** should be used with caution in patients with hepatic damage because it is extensively biotransformed in the liver.
4. the major use of **verapamil** is against supraventricular tachycardia.
5. blockers of calcium channels or of β-adrenoceptors are more effective against dysrhythmias of atrial than of ventricular origin.

Verapamil (a calcium channel blocker) may be given as an antidysrhythmic drug either p.o. (though bioavailability is only about 20%) or i.v. It is extensively metabolized in the liver (half-life about 7 h) and therefore must be used cautiously in patients with severe liver malfunction, otherwise toxic levels may accumulate in the plasma. Because it affects calcium fluxes, its action is more marked in tissues firing frequently such as sinoatrial (SA) and atrioventricular (AV) nodal tissue. The major indication for its use is in supraventricular tachycardias, when it may convert atrial fibrillation and flutter into normal sinus rhythm. **Verapamil** also reduces ventricular rate in atrial disturbances, but is not very effective in dysrhythmias which originate in the ventricles.

The β-adrenoceptor blocking drugs possess, in varying degrees, selectivity for β_1-adrenoceptors, partial agonist activity (intrinsic sympathomimetic activity) and membrane-stabilizing (local anaesthetic) activity. It is clear that the ability to block cardiac β-adrenoceptors confers antidysrhythmic activity, but there may be a contribution from membrane stabilization. The β-adrenoceptor blockers are well tolerated (having wide application as antihypertensive and antianginal drugs). They appear to reduce the incidence of further infarctions and sudden death in patients recovering from acute myocardial infarction, but are less effective in suppressing ventricular ectopic foci than are the sodium channel blockers like **quinidine**.

Paradoxically, cardiac glycosides, like **digoxin**, may be employed as antidysrhythmic agents despite the fact that they may cause dysrhythmias in higher doses. They are used against atrial tachycardias and may convert atrial flutter to fibrillation. Alone, they will not reduce fibrillation but, by depressing AV conduction, they reduce the shower of impulses which would otherwise go on to excite the ventricular muscle. Thus the glycosides can produce a slower, stronger beat from ventricles previously exhibiting tachycardia. Less frequently used nowadays is a combination of **quinidine** and cardiac glycosides (the latter to counteract the atropinic effect of **quinidine**, which sometimes led to ventricular tachycardia). TTTTT

In congestive heart failure

1. the primary cause is the failure of the kidney to excrete sodium.
2. there is usually bradycardia through increased efferent vagal activity.
3. treatment with cardiac glycosides increases ventricular stroke volume.
4. vasodilator drugs like **glyceryl trinitrate** may successfully be used.
5. the heart undergoes hypertrophy in the long term and therefore stroke volume becomes larger than normal.

For more than 200 years, extracts of foxglove (*Digitalis purpurea*) have been known to cure 'dropsy', nowadays called congestive heart failure. The many cardiovascular changes in congestive heart failure are attributable to a reduced contractile capacity of the ventricles for which the system attempts to compensate. Stroke volume is smaller because of the reduced contractions. In an attempt to restore cardiac output, the end-diastolic volume increases (by Starling's law this should increase cardiac force) and venous pressure rises. In addition, sympathetic nervous activity is increased, causing tachycardia and arteriolar vasoconstriction. The resulting increased peripheral resistance leads to decreased renal blood flow and glomerular filtration, which in turn causes more aldosterone to be secreted. The upshot is sodium retention and oedema. Chronically, the heart becomes very enlarged (ventricular hypertrophy) in order to *maintain* stroke volume.

It is possible to treat congestive heart failure with drugs acting at any of three major sites: (a) heart, (b) kidney or (c) peripheral blood vessels. An increased force of contraction (especially in the hypodynamic – or 'failing' – heart) could reverse the cycle of changes described above. With increased cardiac output, activity in the sympathetic system will be reduced, causing heart rate and blood pressure to fall. As the circulation improves, so renal blood flow increases, aldosterone levels fall and retained sodium and water will be excreted. Thus oedema is relieved and peripheral resistance ('after-load') decreased, thereby reducing the work of the heart. Cardiac glycosides (e.g. **digoxin**) are the most important cardiotonic agents, but their therapeutic index is low and toxicity is common. Alternatives have been sought with little success. However, **dopamine**, **dobutamine** (β-adrenoceptor agonist) and **amrinone** (a phosphodiesterase inhibitor) have been used.

By increasing Na^+ and water excretion, thereby reducing oedema, diuretic drugs can bring about improvements in the condition of patients with heart failure, either being used alone or combined with cardiac glycosides.

More attention is being paid to the use of vasodilator drugs in this condition. Drugs which act on the resistance vessels reduce the 'after-load' on the heart, allowing it to work more efficiently (e.g. dihydropyridine Ca^{2+} entry blockers; inhibitors of angiotensin-converting enzyme). Some rapidly acting drugs like **nitroprusside** or **glyceryl trinitrate** also cause venodilation and reduce the 'pre-load'. They are useful in treating acute episodes of heart failure. FFTTF

MCQ 95

The management of chronic congestive heart failure

1. is likely to begin by limiting physical exercise and reducing body weight and salt intake.
2. may involve the use of a thiazide diuretic alone if oedema is pronounced and normal sinus rhythm is present.
3. may require administration of **digoxin** together with a diuretic to enhance excretion of the potassium lost from ventricular cells.
4. may include the use of vasodilator drugs like **hydrallazine** or **prazosin** if other measures do not produce cardiac compensation.
5. is independent of a knowledge of its cause.

Before congestive heart failure can be properly treated, its cause should be identified since it might be due to

(a) mechanical overload (e.g. hypertension, aortic stenosis);
(b) myocardial failure;
(c) pericardial disease.

Only in myocardial failure will drugs such as the cardiac glycosides be effective. Management should begin with an assessment of the patient's history and life-style. A reduction in workload on the heart is essential and can be brought about by limiting physical activity, reducing weight, controlling hypertension, restricting salt and water intake or by any combination of these. Although cardiac glycosides have been the drugs of first choice for decades, it is now increasingly common for therapy to begin with diuretics, especially if oedema is marked and normal sinoatrial nodal rhythm is present.

Thiazide diuretics, like **chlorothiazide**, are now the first choice (as in the treatment of hypertension). Care must be taken to check plasma electrolytes because more potassium is excreted and, if **digitalis** should later be given, its toxicity will be increased during hypokalaemia. **Frusemide** and **ethacrynic acid** produce similar effects and potassium supplements may be necessary. A potassium-sparing diuretic (e.g. **spironolactone**) is occasionally used as an alternative.

Cardiac glycosides (**digoxin** is the most commonly used) are especially useful if cardiac rhythm is disturbed, for example by atrial flutter. However, glycosides give demonstrable relief to only about half the patients with congestive failure and normal rhythm; they are dangerous drugs whose optimal dosage is difficult to estimate. They may be given alone or in combination with diuretics.

Vasodilator drugs are being used increasingly in the treatment of congestive heart failure and are especially helpful in that minority of patients in whom cardiac compensation has not occurred. For example, in patients with concurrent high venous pressure and dyspnoea, nitrates may help (e.g. **isosorbide dinitrate** p.o.). In mechanical overload, presenting the danger of left ventricular failure, drugs selectively dilating arterioles (e.g. **hydrallazine** or a Ca^{2+} entry blocker like **nifedipine**) may be preferred although alternatives like **prazosin** or **phenoxybenzamine** exist which dilate both arteries and veins. Much attention is being paid to inhibitors of angiotensin II formation (inhibitors of angiotensin-converting enzyme, e.g. **captopril**, **enalapril**); their beneficial actions include dilatation of all vessels, as well as increased renal excretion of Na^+ and water because of improved renal flow and the reduced secretion of aldosterone. TTFTF

The cardiac glycosides

1. are all naturally occurring steroidal substances.
2. are chemically a combination of sugars with an aglycone.
3. include **digoxin** and **ouabain**.
4. used clinically all have a long plasma half-life (>48 h).
5. produce initially nausea and vomiting in overdose.

Glycosides are substances formed from one or more sugar molecules combined with another material called an aglycone (or genin). In cardiac glycosides the aglycone is a steroid molecule which has a lactone ring attached at carbon 17. This lactone ring is essential for pharmacological activity as are the hydroxyl groups found in various positions on the steroid rings. The different sugars modify the water solubility and may facilitate absorption and binding of the drugs to cardiac muscle. It has been suggested that the sugar residues might protect the aglycones against enzymes which would otherwise inactivate them.

Three glycosides illustrate the properties of the group as a whole: **digitoxin**, whose aglycone is linked to three molecules of digitoxose; **digoxin**, differing only by possessing one extra −OH group on carbon 12 of the steroid; and **ouabain**, which has only one sugar molecule (rhamnose) but four additional −OH groups on the steroid rings. **Digitoxin** is the most lipid-soluble and best absorbed from the gut. It is highly protein bound and has a long half-life (*nearly 7 days*) so care must be taken to prevent cumulation. Renal impairment scarcely affects the half-life but it may be reduced by drugs that induce liver enzymes. By contrast, **ouabain** is highly polar, not well absorbed from the gut and is given i.v. It is neither bound to plasma proteins nor metabolized and has a half-life of just under 24 h. **Digoxin** is intermediate in its properties but is generally given p.o. at a maintenance dose of about 0.5 mg daily. Care must be taken with **digoxin** (and **ouabain**) in patients with renal failure, where cumulation is especially likely.

Preparations of **digoxin** from different pharmaceutical companies must now fulfil certain requirements with regard to their dissolution rates since the bioavailability was found to be markedly different in formulations from different manufacturers. A change occurred in the bioavailability of **digoxin** from one particular formulation when the manufacturing process was changed, causing many patients, stabilized on the former preparation, to suffer from overdose. The situation was particularly serious because of the low therapeutic index of **digoxin**.

Initial signs of toxicity due to the glycosides are nausea, vomiting, abdominal pain and headache. Serious signs are cardiac dysrhythmias like atrial tachycardia, heart block or ventricular extrasystoles. Death from poisoning occurs by ventricular fibrillation. TTTFT

The action of cardiac glycosides

1. on the failing heart correlates with increased (Na⁺, K⁺)-ATPase activity.
2. in causing a positive inotropic effect is associated with an increase in free Ca^{2+} in ventricular muscle cells.
3. when given to patients with congestive heart failure is to cause tachycardia primarily through increased sympathetic activity.
4. when used to treat disorders of atrial automaticity is to convert atrial fibrillation to atrial flutter.
5. on ventricular automaticity is enhanced when intracellular potassium levels fall.

Cardiac glycosides (**digitoxin, digoxin, ouabain**) cause increased force of contraction in the failing heart. Their mode of action is uncertain, but the increased inotropism correlates with inhibition of (Na⁺, K⁺)-ATPase (the 'sodium pump'). A similar enzyme in skeletal muscle can also be inhibited. Increased inotropic activity is also associated with an increase in the availability of intracellular Ca^{2+}. Most probably these two effects are linked. For instance, removal of excess Ca^{2+} from inside the cardiac muscle cell occurs by some Ca^{2+} being bound to the sarcoplasmic reticulum and by some leaving the cell by exchanging with Na⁺ on the transport mechanism. Thus an inhibition of the sodium pump by glycosides would reduce the rate of exchange of Na⁺ and Ca^{2+}, thereby leaving more Ca^{2+} within the cell. Since free Ca^{2+} is required in the sliding of actin and myosin filaments during muscle shortening, the extra amount could contribute to the increased force of muscle contraction.

The glycosides affect electrical as well as mechanical properties of cardiac muscle, having direct and indirect actions. The refractory period of atrial muscle is shortened; usually a bradycardia occurs and this is intensified by increased vagal activity. Signs of toxicity may appear because the glycosides increase automaticity, sometimes to the extent of causing atrial fibrillation. This property can be turned to clinical advantage in the treatment of atrial flutter (a rapid but coordinated atrial contraction as distinct from the uncoordinated activity in fibrillation). Cardiac glycosides are successful because, although atrial fibrillation results, the showers of impulses from the atria are not transmitted to the ventricles since the glycosides increase the refractory period of the slowly conducting atrioventricular (AV) node. Thus the rapid and irregular *ventricular* beat seen in atrial flutter is converted to a slower regular beat as the AV node takes over as effective pacemaker.

The ventricles respond with increased automaticity, so abnormal rhythms and premature depolarization may occur. Progressive toxicity is revealed by ventricular tachycardia and death will almost certainly occur if ventricular fibrillation sets in. Toxicity is enhanced by the loss of intracellular K⁺ and it is especially important if diuretics (e.g. **chlorothiazide**) are concurrently given to be aware of the possibility of hypokalaemia. Dietary potassium supplements may be necessary. FTFFT

Pharmacology of Blood

MCQ 98

Anaemia

1. may be caused by haemorrhage.
2. of the megaloblastic type can result from a deficiency of **iron**.
3. along with neurological damage is associated with folic acid deficiency.
4. is a consequence of inhibiting DNA synthesis in bone marrow cells.
5. may be caused by toxic cobalt-containing substances known as 'cobalamins'.

Anaemia is a qualitative or quantitative deficiency of red blood cells and results in an inadequate supply of oxygen to the tissues. The oxygen molecules entering the blood through the pulmonary alveoli combine with the red-coloured iron-containing blood pigment haemoglobin (Hb) contained in erythrocytes and are carried to the tissues by the circulation. Anaemia will result if there is suppression of Hb synthesis or of erythrocyte production. **Iron** deficiency states, which may be caused by malabsorption or inadequate diet, reduce Hb production and give rise to microcytic hypochromic anaemia (small erythrocytes with little Hb). If DNA synthesis is inhibited, mitotic activity in erythrocyte stem cells is reduced, causing megaloblastic anaemia (small number of large erythrocytes). This may result from a deficiency of vitamin B_{12} or folic acid, both of which have vital roles in DNA production in the bone marrow, where erythrocytes are made.

Iron is available widely in the diet, especially from meat protein as Hb and myoglobin from which it can be absorbed directly as the Fe^{3+} (ferric) form of haem. In other forms **iron** must first be converted into the Fe^{2+} (ferrous) form in the gut lumen in order to be actively transported into mucosal cells. There it is converted into Fe^{3+} and stored as ferritin or transported out in the form of transferritin to be taken to the bone marrow for Hb synthesis.

Vitamin B_{12} (found in meat, eggs and dairy products) is a group of substances, the cobalamins, which differ according to the chemical groups bound to the central cobalt atom. Some, including **hydroxycobalamin** which is used therapeutically, must be converted to the methyl or the desoxyadenosyl form before they are active in man. The methyl form catalyses the regeneration of tetrahydrofolate from methyl tetrahydrofolate. Without B_{12}, tetrahydrofolate stores diminish and production of purine and pyrimidine nucleotides is halted, thereby inhibiting DNA synthesis and mitosis. Vitamin B_{12} deficiency also results in neurological damage, thought to occur because the desoxyadenosyl form is necessary for the incorporation of vital fatty acids into neuronal membranes.

Folic acid (another of the B vitamins) is found in liver, yeast and spinach and is converted to dihydrofolate and then tetrahydrofolate in cells. The latter is a crucial carrier of one-carbon fragments for synthesis of various nucleosides and amino acids essential for DNA production. TFFTF

For the effective treatment of anaemia

1. its cause must be known.
2. **folic acid** must not be used in vitamin B$_{12}$ deficiency.
3. of the microcytic type, **vitamin B$_{12}$** should be given.
4. due to iron deficiency, **ferrous salts** may have to be given orally for several months.
5. any of the usual remedies may be administered parenterally without untoward effect if a rapid action is necessary.

Anaemias are frequently caused by deficiencies in iron, folic acid or vitamin B$_{12}$ and can be remedied by making good the *particular* deficiency. In microcytic hypochromic anaemia, levels of transferritin in mucosal cells are increased and those of ferritin decreased and this tends to promote the passage of iron to the bone marrow rather than its storage in mucosal cells. Those in whom demand for **iron** is high (premature infants, rapidly growing children and pregnant women) are the most likely to develop **iron** deficiency anaemia though the commonest cause is haemorrhage (e.g. chronic blood loss from gastric ulcers or gut cancer). Oral therapy with **ferrous sulphate** (**fumarate** or **gluconate** being more expensive and of dubious superiority) may be needed for several months to restore normal iron levels. Undesirable effects are usually confined to the gut (e.g. nausea, constipation, abdominal pain) and the black stools produced may make a continuing blood loss (which also produces black stools) less obvious. Acute toxicity in adults is rare, but children are particularly at risk because of the attraction of the bright red shiny pills. Vomiting and diarrhoea result, followed by shock, coma and metabolic acidosis. Specific treatment may involve aspiration of the stomach contents and administration of the iron-chelating compound **deferoxamine.**

For patients who cannot absorb enough iron from the gut, **iron dextran** (*not* ionized iron, which precipitates protein) may be given by i.v. infusion or deep i.m. injections but fever and anaphylactic reactions have resulted and parenteral therapy should only be used if essential.

In megaloblastic anaemias it is important to differentiate between vitamin B$_{12}$ and folic acid deficiency. Although folic acid will improve the blood picture in B$_{12}$ deficiency (since ultimately the condition is caused by a shortage of tetrahydrofolate), the use of folic acid will *not* reverse the neurological damage resulting from B$_{12}$ deficiency and may exacerbate the condition. Only the administration of **Vitamin B$_{12}$** itself will reverse this abnormality.

Vitamin B$_{12}$ deficiency is usually caused by malabsorption (often due to lack of 'intrinsic factor', a glycoprotein from the gastric mucosa which complexes with and permits absorption of B$_{12}$). Therefore therapy is usually parenteral (i.m. injections usually being given monthly for life). Folate deficiency is almost always due to poor diet and cure will occur within weeks with oral **folic acid.** TTFTF

MCQ 100

The coagulation of blood

1. requires the presence of platelets.
2. culminates in the formation of a protein polymer called thrombin, which enmeshes damaged cells.
3. involves the activation, one after another, of pro-enzymes, many of which are synthesized in the liver.
4. occurs slowly in haemophiliacs because of the presence of enzyme inhibitors in the plasma.
5. may be initiated through the intrinsic pathway in the absence of 'tissue factor'.

Complex processes protect the body after traumatic injury and enable the blood to clot, thus plugging damaged vessels and preventing further haemorrhage. Disorders of these processes may lead to failure to terminate trivial or severe haemorrhage. Alternatively, other disorders may lead to coagulation of blood within normal vessels, thus reducing the local blood supply.

The normal coagulation factors found in blood are pro-enzymes synthesized mainly in the liver, which are activated one after another in the sequence shown below, eventually to produce a polymer (fibrin) which sticks to damaged vessels and circulating cells, thereby blocking the leak. The clotting process begins in the intrinsic or extrinsic pathways (each initiated by different factors), which converge on factor X and convert it to its activated form, Xa, the principal activator of prothrombin in the presence of Ca^{2+}. Note that the haemophilias are a group of bleeding disorders caused by a congenital absence of certain factors, like VIII in type A and IX (Christmas factor) in type B haemophilia.

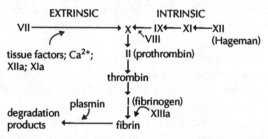

Both blood platelets and the endothelial cells lining vessels have regulatory effects on the coagulation processes. Platelets adhere to damaged cells and aggregate to form a mass which can occlude a vessel and increase the rate of fibrin formation. In the formation of arterial thrombi, platelets aggregate and the adjoining blood vessels constrict under the influence of thromboxane A_2, an arachidonic acid metabolite formed by the platelets themselves. Endothelial cells tend to resist the adhesion of fibrin or platelets to their surface and also produce an arachidonic acid metabolite (prostacyclin; PGI_2) which dilates vessels and opposes the platelet aggregating effect of thromboxane A_2.

The coagulation system (producing fibrin) is in balance with a separate fibrinolytic system which, by production of an enzyme, plasmin, is able to digest fibrin. Excessive clotting can therefore take place because of *over*activity of the coagulation system or *under*activity of the fibrinolytic system. FFTFT

Therapeutically useful anticoagulant drugs

1. may be able to inhibit clotting both *in vivo* and *in vitro*.
2. should not be given by mouth because they cause intestinal bleeding.
3. like the coumarins act by inhibiting vitamin K-dependent production of clotting factors.
4. like **warfarin** are not immediately effective and many days of therapy are needed to achieve a steady-state effect.
5. include **warfarin**, whose activity is enhanced in the presence of drugs like **metronidazole** or sulphonamides.

Various drugs influence the clotting process, some working both *in vitro* and *in vivo* (e.g. **heparin**). Others act only *in vivo*, for example the 'oral anticoagulants' belonging chemically to the coumarin or indanedione groups. The activity of coumarins was discovered when one of them (**dicoumarol**) was identified as the contaminant of sweet clover which had caused haemorrhage in cattle. Several synthetic coumarins are available for clinical use (for example in thrombosis) and all act through the same mechanism. **Warfarin** is the most common (and is also used as a rat poison).

Warfarin acts on the liver to reduce the synthesis of several clotting factors, including prothrombin. All these factors contain carboxyl groups arising from the carboxylation of glutamate residues, under the influence of vitamin K, which permit the binding of Ca^{2+} which is essential for activity. **Warfarin** inhibits the effect of vitamin K; the resulting factors lack carboxyl groups and are inactive. Excess vitamin K can overcome the effect of **warfarin**.

Warfarin is usually given by mouth and its anticoagulant effect appears within a week, though previously synthesized factors (with half-lives from 6 to 60 h) must first be cleared from the plasma before a steady-state effect occurs. **Warfarin** crosses the placenta and should be given only if essential during pregnancy as damaging haemorrhage may occur in the foetus. Also, in the first trimester, the drug may cause abnormal bone development. Many interactions occur between **warfarin** and other drugs. For instance, its actions are enhanced if its biotransformation is blocked (e.g. by **cimetidine** or **metronidazole**); if there is reduced absorption of vitamin K (e.g. in the presence of broad-spectrum antibacterial drugs which decrease bacterial production of vitamin K in the gut); or if it is displaced from its extensive binding to plasma proteins (e.g. by **indomethacin** or sulphonamides). Careful monitoring of coagulation, by measuring prothrombin time, is essential for optimal therapy.

Other vitamin K antagonists are rarely used clinically because they have no advantage over **warfarin**. The indanediones, for example, have been reported to have serious effects on liver and kidney and are implicated in allergic reactions.

While anticoagulant drugs are used as prophylactic measures to reduce the likelihood of clotting, there are occasions (e.g. in treating established thromboses in arteries and veins) when fibrinolytic therapy is required. Fibrinolysis is brought about by a protease, plasmin, formed from inactive plasminogen. **Streptokinase** and **urokinase** are both plasminogen activators but act by different mechanisms. A new (and expensive) fibrinolytic drug, called **eminase**, is reputed to be effective after a single injection in treating myocardial infarction. TFTTT

Heparin

1. is used to prevent recurrent thromboses or postoperatively to reduce venous thromboses.
2. therapy must begin several days before surgery since its anticoagulant effect is delayed.
3. is not absorbed from the gut and must be given parenterally.
4. can be neutralized by the administration of the basic peptide **dextran**.
5. cannot dissolve pre-existing thrombi.

Heparin is used to prevent recurrent thromboses and to reduce the chances of venous thromboses, especially in middle-aged patients after surgery. It is a naturally occurring sulphated acidic polysaccharide, usually obtained from bovine lung or porcine intestine. It is present in mast cell granules, where it binds molecules of histamine. **Heparin** inhibits the coagulation process both *in vivo* and *in vitro* by increasing the ability of a natural protease inhibitor (antithrombin III) to neutralize thrombin and some other clotting factors. The rate at which thrombin is neutralized may be increased by up to 1000-fold by **heparin**.

Heparin must be given parenterally (usually i.v. by infusion or injection) because it cannot be absorbed from the gut. Its action is immediate, lasts for 2–4 h and is terminated by liver heparinase. In addition to its anticoagulant effect, **heparin**, also releases a lipase into the bloodstream which hydrolyses triglycerides to free fatty acids and may also reduce the platelet count. Should the anticoagulant effect of **heparin** need to be terminated, it can be immediately reversed by administration of the basic peptide **protamine sulphate**.

Dextran, a branched polysaccharide, is used as a plasma volume expander in shock or haemorrhage. In its higher molecular weight forms (70 000–75 000 daltons) it can also be used as an antithrombotic agent, principally to reduce the likelihood of venous thromboses postoperatively. Its mechanism of action is unknown though platelet function and fibrin production are depressed.

Fibrinolytic agents act *after* coagulation has occurred. Not only will they cause the lysis of a thrombus which has already formed in an intact vessel, but also they will break down clots that have formed to protect against bleeding from damaged vessels. Fibrinolysis is caused by **streptokinase** and **urokinase** because they activate plasminogen to form plasmin (fibrinolysin), which will dissolve clots. **Eminase** is a new fibrinolytic agent, used in cases of myocardial infarction and reputedly effective after a single injection. These drugs are generally given by i.v. infusion to treat pulmonary embolism. Haemorrhage is the danger during this therapy but can be controlled by giving fibrinogen together with **aminocaproic acid**, which inhibits plasmin formation. **Tranexamic acid** may be substituted for its analogue, **aminocaproic acid**, having a similar mode of action and the same indications for use. TFTFT

Blood platelets

1. can contribute to coagulation processes by releasing fibrinolytic agents.
2. aggregate when exposed to **prostacyclin**.
3. release thromboxane A_2 (a metabolite of arachidonic acid) whose synthesis can be blocked by **aspirin**.
4. exposed to **aspirin** will be permanently damaged because they cannot synthesize replacement cyclo-oxygenase.
5. aggregate more readily in the presence of **imidazole**.

Blood platelets contribute to the clotting process by aggregating and thus plugging damaged vessels. Many substances promote aggregation (collagen, adrenaline) but the arachidonic acid metabolite thromboxane A_2 (TxA_2) produced by the platelets themselves is the most potent pro-aggregatory agent known.

Drugs which can inhibit aggregation are potentially useful in patients at risk from the production of intra-arterial thrombi. **Aspirin**, for example, irreversibly acetylates cyclo-oxygenase and prevents platelets forming the endoperoxides, prostaglandins G_2 and H_2, the further metabolism of which forms TxA_2. Since the effect of **aspirin** is irreversible and platelets cannot themselves synthesize cyclo-oxygenase, new platelets must be produced for recovery to take place. There is evidence that the daily dose of **aspirin** prescribed for prophylaxis of thromboembolic disorders (1–1.5 g) is less able to prevent aggregation than expected, probably because vascular endothelial cell cyclo-oxygenase is also blocked, which prevents the production of prostacyclin (PGI_2), a potent natural antagonist of TxA_2. Lower doses of **aspirin** (50 mg daily), given chronically, reduce platelet TxA_2 production by about 90% with little effect on endothelial PGI_2 synthesis and thus may have a net antiaggregatory effect. Other non-steroidal anti-inflammatory drugs also block cyclo-oxygenase.

Imidazole is a TxA_2 synthesis inhibitor which has little effect on PGI_2 production and thus exerts a net antiaggregatory effect, like low doses of **aspirin**. A number of new drugs with similar properties are currently under development for use in the treatment of thrombotic disorders.

Prostacyclin itself has a half-life of a few minutes but is used to inhibit platelet aggregation in extracorporeal circulations (e.g. during haemodialysis and in heart–lung machines). It is usually given by continuous infusion into the extracorporeal blood and little of the administered dose gets back into the vascular system.

The precursor of prostaglandins and thromboxanes is arachidonic acid, formed by the action of phospholipase A_2 on membrane phospholipids. In addition to arachidonate, this reaction can also produce platelet activating factor (PAF; acetyl-glyceryl-ether-phosphorylcholine) via an intermediate called lyso-PAF, which requires acetylation for the conversion. Production of PAF should be expected in circumstances when prostaglandins are abundantly formed, since it is generated by most types of inflammatory cells (polymorphonuclear leucocytes, macrophages, basophils and platelets

continued on next page 127

themselves). Platelet activating factor induces a change in platelet shape and promotes release of the contents of platelet granules, thus initiating and contributing to aggregation. It has a variety of other pro-inflammatory actions including vasodilatation, increased vascular permeability, hyper-algesia, bronchoconstriction, and chemotaxis of leucocytes. Antagonists of PAF are being sought, which may be useful against some inflammatory conditions. It should be noted that PAF synthesis is blocked by *steroidal* but not by non-steroidal anti-inflammatory drugs. FFTTF

Bleeding disorders

1. may be inherited, as with haemophilias type A and B.
2. due to a lack of factor VIII are best treated with **vitamin K**.
3. due to severe liver failure cannot be corrected by administration of **vitamin K**.
4. may respond to **aminocaproic acid** if they are caused by fibrinolytic therapy with **streptokinase**.
5. will be cured by the administration of the missing coagulation factor (**urokinase** in haemophilia type A, for example).

Several coagulation disorders have a genetic basis and in most of these a particular clotting factor is absent or in short supply. Haemophilia A (factor VIII deficiency) or B (factor IX deficiency) are the most common (95% of cases). Both these coagulation factors are available as concentrated human plasma fractions and are given by i.v. infusion at times when patients are particularly at risk. For instance, factor VIII will be intermittently infused to give levels 5–15% of normal for periods of 1–5 days to treat uncontrolled bleeding into joints. For surgery or major trauma, levels two or three times higher may be needed for at least a week. With this type of clotting disorder it is not the major haemorrhage which is the main problem but the minor continuing blood loss (bruising, for example), which causes pain and disability. As with all blood products derived from human sources, clotting factors, when administered, may introduce blood-borne diseases, although the future production of clotting factors using genetically engineered organisms may alleviate this problem.

Most coagulation factors are synthesized in the liver, which is why hepatic failure may lead to the development of bleeding disorders. Such disorders are not relieved by **vitamin K** administration, though some inherited disorders may be.

Vitamin K is found in liver, egg yolk and many vegetable oils but a large proportion of that available to the body is synthesized in the gut by luminal bacteria. Bile salts are normally essential for its absorption, but water-soluble derivatives of the vitamin are available for therapeutic use which do not require their presence. Plasma levels of clotting factors begin to rise about 6 h after administration of **vitamin K**. It is often given to neonates who may be deficient in **vitamin K** during the perinatal period.

An adjunct in the treatment of haemophilia is **aminocaproic acid**. It is an orally active inhibitor of fibrinolysis, preventing the activation of plasminogen (and hence production of the fibrinolytic plasmin). It is also used to treat bleeding which occurs during fibrinolytic therapy with **streptokinase** or **urokinase**. Major unwanted effects are hypotension, diarrhoea and nasal stuffiness. Rare, but potentially dangerous, is the development of intravascular thrombi due to a reduction in the normal plasmin levels. TFTTF

Autacoids
and
Allergy

Allergic reactions

1. have an immunological basis and therefore only occur in the presence of circulating antibodies.
2. are either 'immediate' or 'delayed' according to the time elapsing between the first (sensitizing) and second (challenge) antigen exposure.
3. of types I, II and III are mediated by antibodies of the IgE group of immunoglobulins.
4. of type IV are associated with lymphokines, released from sensitized T-lymphocytes.
5. affect target cells which differ according to animal species.

Allergies are undesirable reactions brought about by exposure to chemical substances in doses which would normally be innocuous. The allergic state has an immunological basis, so the biological processes are similar to the defence mechanisms normally associated with the immune system. An allergic reaction can only occur on the second or later exposure to the provocative chemical itself (called the allergen or antigen) or a closely related material (cross-allergy). Typically, on the first (sensitizing) contact no overt changes occur but the chemical structure would have been perceived as 'foreign' and the immune process activated. Consequently, about 2–3 weeks later, the blood would contain high levels of lymphocytes (B- or T-cells) which have special features that enable them to recognize the antigen should they meet it again.

The B-lymphocytes are precursors of 'plasma cells' which are secretory, their products being proteins called immunoglobulins (Ig; five separate classes are known, A, D, E, G and M, with molecular weights of 165 000–900 000 daltons). Immunoglobulin molecules are antibodies and so will bind selectively to the antigen that evoked their synthesis. Large amounts are found in the bloodstream and some (IgE especially) become firmly fixed to receptors on target cells. When antigen and its specific IgE counterpart bind together, the union triggers a cascade of events culminating in an 'immediate' allergic reaction, so-called because it takes place within minutes of the binding. Immediate reactions are divided into three categories: *type I* (allergen binding to IgE), which results in a release of biologically active substances from the target mast cells; *type II*, where antibodies are directed towards cell surface proteins, binding to which results in cytolysis and cell death; *type III*, in which usually IgG reacts with antigen in the bloodstream to form a soluble complex that then damages blood-vessel walls.

T-Lymphocytes do not secrete Ig molecules. Instead, antigens interact with receptors on the surface of the T-cells. This triggers a release of macromolecules (lymphokines) from the T-cell. Some lymphokines are chemotactic and others mitogenic or cytotoxic and these properties are responsible for the *type IV* reactions. Since these events take hours or even days to develop after antigen gains access to the body, they are described as 'delayed' hypersensitivity reactions. FFFTT

MCQ 106

Immunoglobulins

1. are bilaterally symmetrical proteins.
2. can be split by proteolytic enzymes into dissimilar fragments with distinct biological properties.
3. are divided into five groups (A, D, E, G and M) based on physicochemical properties.
4. include reaginic antibody, which has a longer half-life when fixed to its target cell than when free in the circulation.
5. are placed in different classes to signify that each class reacts with different antigens.

Type I is the most common of the 'immediate' allergic hypersensitivity reactions. It is triggered when allergen binds to antibody (usually immunoglobulin (IgE) that has already circulated and become fixed to the target cell surface. These antibodies possess two distinct binding sites, one for the acceptor on the cell surface and one for the allergen. Each highly coiled Ig molecule consists of two pairs of amino acid chains (L = light and H = heavy), joined by disulphide bridges to form a bilaterally symmetrical structure. Certain proteolytic enzymes (papain and pepsin) cleave the Ig molecules in specific positions to produce protein fragments which still retain biological activity. One such, the F_c fragment, is able to bind to the acceptor site on the target cell surface. Another, the F_{ab} fragment, binds selectively to antigen molecules.

The five types of Ig (A, D, E, G and M) vary in physicochemical properties and biological functions but, importantly, differ from each other in the amino acid sequences of their H chains. Since the H chains determine the F_c structure, the differences permit IgE to bind to acceptors on the mast cell surface but other Ig types to bind less readily because their peptide sequences (and hence three-dimensional structures) are different.

The geometry of the F_{ab} fragment is determined by the amino acid sequence in the L chain, changes in which govern the specificity of the antibody. Since identical sequences may be found in the L chain of IgE and IgG molecules within the same animal, this explains how antibodies from different classes can bind to a common antigen.

The term 'reaginic' antibody is often used synonymously with IgE and draws attention to the highly reactive nature of this protein. Compared with other Ig types, reaginic antibody is heat-labile (like complement it is inactivated by heating to 56 °C for an hour), is present in serum in very low concentrations and has a high affinity for mast cell acceptors. It remains fixed to the acceptors for periods greater than 10 days, during which time the cells are said to be sensitized because the antibody can bind antigen. The half-life of IgE is much shorter when this antibody is circulating in the bloodstream. TTTTF

The substances to which an organism becomes allergic

1. must be proteins or chemicals capable of binding to proteins.
2. are called haptens if they need to be chemically bound to a larger molecule to make them antigenic.
3. can evoke a release of chemical mediators if added to appropriately sensitized isolated tissue.
4. when introduced for the first time to an animal may cause passive sensitization.
5. will cause isolated ileum to contract if the tissue is taken from a guinea-pig previously sensitized to the same substance.

Antigen is a term which describes any material that can bring about a specific immunological response *in vivo* or *in vitro*. Substances with minimum molecular weights (MWs) of about 1000 daltons (e.g. oxytocin, angiotensin) may stimulate lymphocytes to produce antibodies but, generally, the higher the MW, the more immunogenic the substance. Not only proteins but also carbohydrates are immunogenic (if the MW is greater than 100 000 daltons). Animal proteins (in excreta, scales, fur) and plant pollens frequently act as antigens.

Allergy may develop to drugs that have a low MW. Small molecules with antigenic properties are called haptens. Alone they could not evoke antibody production but by chemically combining with a protein in plasma or skin, for instance, they may sufficiently alter the three-dimensional structure of the protein to make it appear foreign. The resulting antibodies will bind either to the modified protein or to the hapten itself because their L chains are complementary in structure to the hapten molecules.

The process leading to the production of lymphocytes which recognize a specific antigen is known as active sensitization. However, whole animals and certain of their tissues may be rendered passively sensitized by administering lymphocytes or serum containing antibodies from an actively sensitized donor. In any of these cases an overt allergic reaction should result when the animal (or its sensitized tissue) is challenged with antigen. These biological principles are exploited in the search for antiallergic drugs using, for example:

(a) Schultz–Dale reactions (smooth muscle contractions; active sensitization; type I reaction; usually non-reaginic antibody);
(b) passive cutaneous anaphylactic reactions (skin inflammation; type I reaction; usually reaginic antibody);
(c) anaphylactic reactions in human lung fragments (measuring released chemical mediators; passive sensitization; type I reaction; IgE).

FTTFT

MCQ 108

Type I allergic reactions

1. occur after interaction of antigen and IgE in human lung tissue either *in vivo* or *in vitro*.
2. cannot be brought about in passively sensitized tissues.
3. resemble closely the effects of peptides like bradykinin which are released from sensitized mast cells.
4. can be suppressed by drugs which antagonize the effects of adrenal medullary amines.
5. are associated with increased extracellular levels of histamine and of arachidonic acid metabolites such as leukotrienes.

During surgery for lung cancer, fragments of undamaged lung can be taken from the excised lobes and used in allergy research. The fragments may be sliced thinly or macerated in a blender and, after a washing process, a suspension of the tissue is incubated in serum from an allergic patient. The allergy will be manifested towards a material like house-dust mite or grass pollen. After several hours of incubation the lung mast cells will have become passively sensitized by the IgE antibodies present in the serum. After washing, the lung tissue can now be challenged to elicit a type I reaction. Addition of antigen (soluble mite- or pollen-protein) triggers the release mechanism, causing an accumulation of chemical mediators in the extracellular fluid. The fluid can then be analysed chemically or biologically and this type of experiment can be used to judge if the allergic release reaction can be modified by drugs.

Many substances are liberated from lung tissues during such reactions. Histamine and heparin are liberated from stores in the metachromatic granules of mast cells. Several biologically active products are derived from the phospholipids of cell membranes. They include the eicosanoids, a family of unsaturated lipids with a chain of 20 carbon atoms (e.g. prostaglandins, thromboxanes and leukotrienes); another product is platelet activating factor (acetyl-glyceryl-ether-phosphorylcholine), which acts on platelets and by this and other actions plays an important role in some inflammatory conditions. Unlikely to be released from isolated chopped tissue, but associated with type I reactions *in vivo*, are substances like bradykinin (a nonapeptide derived from an α-globulin found in plasma) and acetylcholine or adrenaline (released from parasympathetic nerves and the adrenal medulla respectively). These materials serve to modulate the developing allergic reaction. By affecting the synthesis, storage, release or the subsequent biological actions of these substances, it should be possible with drugs to alter the extent of allergic reactions. Most drugs employed clinically for their antiallergic activity will have been demonstrated to interact with chemical mediators in these ways. TFFFT

Of the substances released in the course of an immediate allergic reaction

1. both histamine and bradykinin cause peripheral vasoconstriction and bronchoconstriction.
2. leukotrienes and bradykinin are acidic lipids which contain sulphur.
3. acetylcholine is an important bronchoconstrictor substance *in vivo*.
4. adrenaline can produce vasodilatation and bronchodilatation.
5. histamine, leukotrienes and bradykinin will be found in pulmonary venous blood during an asthmatic attack.

Biological and chemical assays show that many different substances are released into the bloodstream during a type I allergic reaction. Which of these materials cause the tissue responses remains to be established. Allergic reactions in the lungs cause:

(a) spasm or increased tone in the airway smooth muscle;
(b) oedema (swelling) of the bronchial mucosa associated with increases in vascular permeability;
(c) the accumulation of bronchial secretions.

All three contribute to the respiratory difficulties characteristic of asthma. Intravenous injection of **histamine** in man brings about the same triad of effects and endogenously released histamine would be expected to act similarly. The cysteinyl-leukotrienes (**LTC$_4$, D$_4$** and **E$_4$**) are potent spasmogens of human isolated bronchial muscle and cause mucous secretion and wheezing in human subjects. Another phospholipid metabolite, **platelet activating factor**, causes bronchoconstriction and pulmonary oedema in several species of laboratory animals. The nonapeptide **bradykinin** dilates peripheral blood vessels, increases vascular permeability and, in guinea-pigs, induces airway smooth muscle contraction. Compared with **histamine**, the bronchoconstrictor effect of **bradykinin** develops more slowly, taking up to several minutes for the maximal effect to be achieved and several minutes to wane after injection in anaesthetized guinea-pigs.

Both acetylcholine and adrenaline will be released secondarily during allergic reactions *in vivo*, either through reflexes or, sometimes, the latter will be released by direct stimulation of adrenal medullary cells by substances like histamine and bradykinin.

Acetylcholine from postganglionic vagal fibres causes bronchoconstriction. Circulating adrenaline is a vasodilator and a bronchodilator substance, thereby functionally antagonizing bronchoconstrictors; it also opposes increases in venular permeability caused by drugs like **histamine**. It seems likely, therefore, that when a type I reaction occurs *in vivo*, its consequences are made less dramatic by the actions of adrenaline, whose release from the adrenal medulla and subsequent circulation to the lungs almost invariably accompanies the first signs of an allergic reaction. FFTTT

MCQ 110

Histamine

1. is biosynthesized by deamination of the amino acid histidine by histidine decarboxylase.
2. is stable enough to resist boiling for several minutes in acid solution.
3. injected intradermally causes a triple response (erythema, oedema and flare).
4. may be bioassayed on guinea-pig or mouse isolated ileum, both of which respond to concentrations in the nanomolar range.
5. produces gastric acid secretion and uterine relaxation by stimulating H_2-receptors.

Histamine (β-imidazolyl ethylamine) is a naturally occurring substance with a wide range of biological actions. It is biosynthesized, mainly in the mast cells found in tissues like skin, lungs, gut etc. and also in some CNS neurones, from the dietary amino acid histidine, which is decarboxylated by histidine decarboxylase with pyridoxal phosphate as a co-factor. Histamine is remarkably stable and is resistant to boiling for several hours in acid solution.

On injection into mammalian skin, **histamine** evokes a 'triple response' (like that seen with nettle stings or after drawing a blunt probe across delicate skin) comprising the following three components:

(a) reddening (erythema);
(b) a weal (oedema);
(c) areas of redness (flare).

Erythema occurs around the injection site due to arteriolar dilatation. Oedema occurs at the centre of the injection caused by leakage of plasma proteins from venules. **Histamine** increases permeability and the escaping proteins draw more water into the extravascular space by osmosis (note that venular *not* capillary permeability is increased). Flare develops at sites several centimetres away from the injection. Flare is caused by a release of vasodilator substances (e.g. substance P) from sensory nerves activated antidromically when **histamine** stimulates terminals of other branches of the same nerves (axon reflex). Stimulation of sensory nerves by **histamine** is responsible for the pain and/or itch which accompanies a nettle sting.

Histamine also causes contraction of intestinal smooth muscle, that of guinea-pig gut being especially sensitive, sometimes responding to concentrations as low as 1×10^{-8} M. By contrast, mouse or rat small intestine may fail to contract even to concentrations 10 000 times higher. A histamine-induced tachycardia (via histamine-sensitive adenylate cyclase) occurs in several species both *in vivo* and *in vitro*. **Histamine** is a powerful secretagogue, acting to release adrenaline from adrenal medullary cells and to release HCl from the oxyntic cells of the stomach mucosa.

Three types of receptor (H_1, H_2 and H_3) mediate the actions of histamine. Most actions on smooth muscles are elicited through H_1 receptors, whilst the important consequences of H_2-receptor activation are gastric acid secretion, tachycardia and, particularly in the rat, uterine muscle relaxation. The H_3-receptors are found in the CNS, for instance on nerve endings in the rat cerebral cortex, where they appear to exert autoinhibitory actions on the release of histamine from these neurones. FTTFT

Antihistamine drugs which block H₁-receptors

1. cause release of adrenal medullary amines.
2. include phenothiazines, like **promethazine**.
3. may be used to treat asthma because they affect airway smooth muscle.
4. have sedative effects.
5. inhibit the formation of eicosanoids.

Antihistamine drugs fall into two major categories, according to whether they block H$_1$- or H$_2$-receptors (although the discovery of an autoinhibitory receptor in the CNS, termed H$_3$-, which can be blocked by e.g. **thioperamide** provides a third group). The classical antihistamines, discovered in the 1930s, act on H$_1$-receptors and, therefore, block the following effects of histamine:

(a) contraction of intestinal smooth muscle;
(b) contraction of bronchial smooth muscle;
(c) the vasodilatation and increased venular permeability to plasma proteins;
(d) pain and itch caused by sensory nerve stimulation;
(e) release of adrenal medullary amines.

Many antihistamines used in hay fever cause drowsiness and users must be cautioned about the additive effects when other CNS depressants are taken in conjunction (especially **alcohol**); tasks demanding fine coordination and alertness must be avoided particularly if, as in driving, mistakes could endanger life. Some newer antihistamines, for example **terfenadine** and **astemizole**, are virtually devoid of sedative effects.

A dry mouth often occurs when antihistamines are taken, the result of atropine-like actions. However, atropinic actions are not always undesirable; such actions on the CNS contribute to the beneficial effect of **promethazine** when used in the prophylaxis of motion sickness.

Despite their effectiveness in hay fever, these antihistamines are ineffective in the treatment of asthma. This is a paradox since human lung tissue sensitized with antibodies that react to pollens (as in hay fever) or to house-dust mite (as in asthma) will release histamine when challenged with the appropriate antigen. It is suggested that other chemical mediators are relatively more important in asthma (e.g. eicosanoids such as leukotrienes). Alternatively, the sites of action and the high local concentration of histamine during asthmatic attacks may hinder the access of antihistamines to the receptor. FTFTF

MCQ 112

Cimetidine *is an example of an antihistaminic drug blocking H₂-receptors*

1. as is **ranitidine**.
2. and will therefore cause relaxation of the rat uterus.
3. which reduces the secretion of gastric acid provoked by efferent vagal stimulation.
4. but has no effect on the tachycardia induced by **histamine.**
5. which is used in the treatment of peptic ulceration.

As well as the classical antihistamines (H_1-blockers) there are antagonists which compete with histamine to block

  (a) gastric acid secretion;
  (b) tachycardia;
  (c) relaxation of the rat uterus.

These three effects are caused by stimulation of H_2-receptors. The existence of this separate group of receptors was confirmed in the 1970s through the study of histamine analogues with varying degrees of selectivity in causing guinea-pig ileum to contract (H_1) or rat oxyntic cells to secrete HCl (H_2). This spurred the development of drugs (based on the structure of histamine) which could block H_2-receptors. First **burimamide**, then **metiamide** and next **cimetidine** were followed by others such as **ranitidine**. These drugs differ in relative potency, in the extent to which they are absorbed from the gut and in possessing other pharmacological actions, some of which may be clinically undesirable. For instance, by blocking androgen receptors, **cimetidine** may cause gynaecomastia (breast enlargement in males). This drug can also inhibit liver mono-oxygenases, thereby reducing the biotransformation of, for example, some benzodiazepines and β-adreno-ceptor blockers; this hepatic effect is potentially dangerous if the metabolism of drugs with a low therapeutic index is reduced (e.g. **warfarin, phenytoin, theophylline**). **Ranitidine** has neither of these actions. The H_2-receptor blockers were designed with one clinical outlet in mind: since they all inhibit gastric acid secretion, they should speed the healing of peptic ulcers or, in susceptible patients, prevent their development. The H_2-receptor blocking drugs have been used very successfully in this area and are now the most widely prescribed drugs for the management of peptic ulcers.

In assessing the action of H_2-receptor blocking drugs, a variety of stimuli can be used in experimental animals to promote gastric acid secretion (e.g. **histamine** itself or an analogue such as **betazole, pentagastrin**, food or stimulation of the efferent vagal nerves to the stomach). In the last-mentioned case the administration of atropine-like drugs inhibits the vagally mediated secretion though atropinics are relatively ineffective against the other stimuli. However, H_2-receptor blockers reduce the effects of all these secretagogues, implying that histamine is involved in a terminal pathway common to all these stimuli. Although atropinic drugs are less effective than H_2-receptor blockers and tend to produce undesirable effects by blocking muscarinic receptors elsewhere in the body, selective blockers

140

continued on next page

are being sought on the basis that several types of muscarinic receptor exist. For instance, **pirenzipine** fairly selectively blocks the M_1-receptors (serving gastric secretion but not the other peripheral muscarinic functions) and therefore has fewer side-effects than other atropinics.

Despite the identification of H_2-receptors in cardiac and uterine tissue, no clinically useful action has yet been claimed for these drugs at these sites. TFTFT

MCQ 113

Of the drugs which are used to treat peptic ulcer

1. **magnesium hydroxide** causes constipation.
2. both **aluminium hydroxide** and **sodium bicarbonate** are absorbed principally from the small intestine.
3. many neutralize free acid and thereby reduce the proteolytic activity of pepsin.
4. **metoclopramide** is also an antiemetic drug which blocks central dopamine receptors.
5. **carbenoxolone**, from liquorice root, has mineralocorticoid activity.

Healing of established peptic ulcers (or prevention of their formation) may be promoted if gastric acidity is reduced. This may be brought about by inhibiting acid secretion, the most effective drugs being histamine H_2-receptor blockers like **cimetidine** and **ranitidine**, while atropinic agents may also be effective, especially if, like **pirenzipine**, they selectively block the muscarinic M_1-receptors on the oxyntic cells. Alternatively, measures can be employed to neutralize the free acid sufficiently to stop its irritant effect on the sensitive mucosa. The damaging effect on ulcerated tissue by pepsin would also be reduced as raising the pH decreases its proteolytic activity.

Some antacids contain poorly absorbed cations (Mg^{2+}, Al^{3+}) and they cannot, therefore, cause systemic alkalosis. However, magnesium chloride formed in the stomach and magnesium carbonate in the small intestine may have a purgative action. The **hydroxides** of **magnesium** and **aluminium** are often given together, as **aluminium** may cause a compensatory constipation, yet both contribute to the pH effect. There has been speculation that senile dementia (Alzheimer's disease) may be associated with a high intake of **aluminium**, but there is no evidence that its use in antacid preparations constitutes a serious risk.

Sodium bicarbonate is frequently used but has many disadvantages. It has a short duration of effect and the CO_2 formed may distend the stomach and cause belching. In cases of kidney dysfunction, systemic alkalosis may occur because HCO_3^- is rapidly absorbed from the small intestine and in some patients the kidney may not be able to respond as quickly as usual to secrete an alkaline urine.

Carbenoxolone accelerates the healing of ulcers when given orally. Its absorption is rapid, it is highly bound to plasma proteins and its glucuronide conjugate enters the enterohepatic circulation via the bile. The major unwanted effects of **carbenoxolone** are due to its mineralocorticoid activity (sodium retention and potassium loss, causing oedema and hypertension). They may need to be countered by diuretics and potassium supplements. Care is needed with the latter, which may aggravate ulcers.

A **bismuth** compound (**tripotassium dicitrate bismuthate, De-Nol**) not only coats the gastric mucosa but stimulates mucus production, binds to pepsin and inhibits microbial activity and gut movements. The substance is not absorbed.

Metoclopramide, a drug with a variety of uses in the gut (including antiemetic, has been reported to promote the healing of ulcers. Its antiemetic action is principally through antagonism of dopamine in the CNS. It also accelerates the passage of material through the gut by enhancing cholinergic mechanisms. FFTTT

Membrane phospholipids may give rise to arachidonic acid metabolites which include

1. thromboxane A_2.
2. leukotrienes.
3. prostaglandins E_1 and E_2.
4. platelet activating factor.
5. 6-keto-prostaglandin $F_{1\alpha}$.

Arachidonic acid (AA; 5,8,11,14-eicosatetraenoic acid) has a chain of 20 carbon atoms ('eicosa' from the Greek for 20; 'tetraen', denoting four double bonds). Provided the chain length is unchanged, all the metabolites are called eicosanoids.

Arachidonic acid occurs as a dietary fatty acid and becomes incorporated into the phospholipids of cell membranes. The enzyme phospholipase A_2 can liberate AA, along with the precursor of platelet activating factor (PAF), lyso-PAF, from the phospholipids. Alternatively, AA but not PAF, can be formed in a two-step reaction begun by phospholipase C. The enzymes cyclo-oxygenase and lipoxygenase then initiate the formation of a variety of products from AA.

Cyclo-oxygenase causes:

(a) the formation of a five-membered ring (carbons 8 and 12 becoming linked);
(b) a rearrangement of double bonds leaving two in the side-chains;
(c) the incorporation of more oxygen atoms in the molecule.

Early workers called some of the products prostaglandins, in the mistaken belief that the prostate gland was their major source, and both this term and its abbreviation PG have been retained. The initial products (cyclic endoperoxides PGG_2 and PGH_2) are rapidly converted by isomerases/reductases to more stable substances like PGD_2, E_2, $F_{2\alpha}$, or by other enzymes to prostacyclin (PGI_2; with a double ring) or to thromboxane A_2 (TxA_2; with a single oxane ring). They all belong to the '2' series for they retain the *two* double bonds from PGG_2. However, 6-keto-$PGF_{1\alpha}$, from which one double bond is lost, is an important metabolite of PGI_2. Other eicosanoic acids (trien- or pentaen-) could substitute for AA and would give rise to the '1' and '3' series of PG respectively.

Alternatively, a lipoxygenase system causes double-bond rearrangements and oxygen incorporation without inducing ring formation in the AA molecule. The products are called leukotrienes (LT). TTFFT

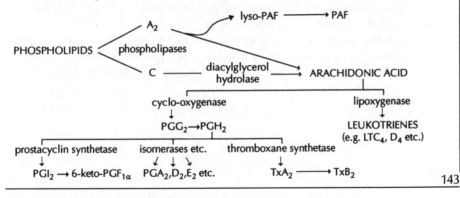

MCQ 115

The biological actions of substances derived from membrane phospholipids include

1. vasoconstriction and platelet aggregation by thromboxane A_2.
2. bronchoconstriction and pulmonary oedema by platelet activating factor.
3. platelet aggregation and bronchodilatation by prostacyclin.
4. contraction of uterine and intestinal smooth muscle by prostaglandin E_2.
5. vasodilatation and bronchodilatation by leukotrienes C_4 and D_4.

A variety of stimuli (mechanical, thermal, chemical) activate the enzyme phospholipase A_2, which liberates (from membrane phospholipids) arachidonic acid as well as the precursor of platelet activating factor (PAF), lyso-PAF. A cascade of products can arise from arachidonic acid, initiated either by cyclo-oxygenation (types of prostaglandin, PG, and thromboxane, Tx) or lipoxygenation (types of leukotriene, LT). Most of the products are biologically active and are thought to play important roles in many bodily processes. All tissues are capable of generating the precursors, though the final products depend on the possession of the particular converting enzymes.

Among the cyclized products are substances with opposing actions. For instance, TxA_2 (liberated from platelets when they contact a foreign surface) causes platelets to aggregate and small vessels to constrict. Its actions are opposed by PGI_2, an antiaggregatory product of vascular endothelial cells which also relaxes most smooth muscles (e.g. vascular, bronchial). Prostaglandin E_2 also dilates airways and blood vessels, but causes contraction of intestinal and gravid uterine muscle, the last action being the basis of its use to induce labour or abortion. Prostaglandin D_2 is produced especially by mast cells in lung tissue, possesses powerful bronchoconstrictor actions and has been implicated as a mediator of human asthma.

Leukotrienes have been detected during, and probably contribute to, inflammatory reactions in many tissues. The cysteinyl-derivatives (LTC_4, D_4 and E_4) contract most smooth muscles and increase vascular permeability. The material called slow-reacting substance of anaphylaxis, discovered five decades ago, is now known to be a mixture of LTC_4, D_4 and E_4.

Platelet activating factor is a recent addition to this list of putative mediators. Produced by a variety of leucocytes, it not only induces shape change and release of chemicals from platelets, but has numerous pro-inflammatory actions including vasodilatation, oedema, bronchoconstriction, leucocyte chemotaxis and hyperalgesia.

Thus, while many of these substances could be regarded individually as an inflammatory mediator, they are more likely to act in concert, thereby making inflammatory processes more difficult to control therapeutically. TTFTF

A vascular perfusate from antigenically challenged lungs may be bioassayed by cascading the fluid over a series of isolated tissues. Such experiments show that

1. eicosanoids are commonly liberated into the fluid during the allergic reaction.
2. **mepyramine** will prevent the allergic reaction from causing a release of histamine.
3. substances are released which cause a contraction of rabbit isolated aorta.
4. **aspirin**, added to the superfusate, blocks the effects of released mediators on the bioassay tissues.
5. non-steroidal anti-inflammatory drugs reduce the output of leuko-trienes.

Eicosanoids, which include metabolites of arachidonic acid from both cyclo-oxygenase and lipoxygenase pathways, produce a large number of biological effects. They may have wide physiological importance because their presence has been detected during many physiological or pathophysiological events and some eicosanoids mimic the events themselves. In many other fields selective antagonists can be used to investigate the functions of endogenous ligands. Few receptor blockers of eicosanoids are available, although development of several can be expected in the near future. However, the biosynthesis of eicosanoids can be blocked by enzyme inhibitors. These have proved to be useful investigative tools and, in many cases, have been known for years as useful drugs though their mechanism of action was only discovered in the 1970s.

Non-steroidal anti-inflammatory drugs (e.g. **aspirin, ibuprofen, indomethacin**) act principally by blocking *cyclo-oxygenation* of arachidonic acid. The production of leukotrienes is unaffected or even increased since it involves the *lipoxygenase* pathway. The key to **aspirin**'s action was discovered in 1969 during experiments which measured the output of chemical mediators from perfused lungs of guinea-pigs. The mediators were measured by bioassay by passing the perfusate over several isolated organ preparations arranged in series. The organs were carefully chosen because of their selectivity in responding to endogenous ligands so that mixtures of active substances could be identified and quantified. In lungs receiving **aspirin**, a particular biologically active substance called RCS (rabbit aorta contracting substance) was no longer liberated. RCS is now known to be thromboxane A_2, or a mixture of thromboxane and cyclic endoperoxides, the constitution differing according to the tissue of origin. This early experiment implied that **aspirin** inhibited the release process, but it is now known to inhibit synthesis; this is tantamount to blocking release in a system where the end-products are synthesized on demand instead of being stored in cells prior to release. **Aspirin** does not block eicosanoid receptors and therefore leaves the tissues free to respond to exogenous material.

Mepyramine does not block the release of mediators but is an antagonist of histamine at H_1-receptors. TFTFF

MCQ 117

Experiments in which the production of eicosanoids by isolated tissues has been measured show that

1. both steroidal and non-steroidal anti-inflammatory drugs block the biosynthesis of leukotrienes.
2. **dexamethasone** inhibits the enzyme lipoxygenase.
3. **indomethacin** prevents the biosynthesis of prostaglandins from endogenous but not exogenous arachidonic acid.
4. drugs like **dexamethasone** are competitive inhibitors of phospholipase A_2.
5. **puromycin** can prevent the inhibitory effects of **dexamethasone**.

Eicosanoids are implicated in the mechanism of action of several groups of drugs, including both steroidal (e.g. **dexamethasone**) and non-steroidal (e.g. **indomethacin**) anti-inflammatory agents. These two groups of drugs resemble each other in reducing inflammation and in producing or aggravating gastric ulceration, but they differ with respect to the enzymes on which they act to produce their effects. For instance, **indomethacin** is a cyclo-oxygenase inhibitor and stops production of all prostaglandins and thromboxanes from exogenous or endogenous arachidonic acid. **Indomethacin** does not block lipoxygenase so the production of leukotrienes is not affected.

By contrast, **dexamethasone** does not inhibit cyclo-oxygenase and does not prevent the production of prostaglandins from exogenous arachidonic acid. It does, however, inhibit the production of prostaglandins in tissues which have to make their own arachidonic acid, by preventing the production of arachidonic acid itself. This acid is formed intracellularly when membrane phospholipids are broken down by an enzyme, phospholipase A_2, located in the plasma membrane. **Dexamethasone** has been shown not to inhibit the enzyme directly but to cause the synthesis and release of a protein which is a potent inhibitor of phospholipase A_2. In order to work, **dexamethasone** is taken up into the target cells and binds to steroid receptors; the drug–receptor complex is then transported to the cell nucleus. Here there is a promotion of RNA-directed synthesis of the inhibitory protein. Several groups of workers have studied the product from different cells and though differences in, for example, molecular weight were reported, an analysis of antienzyme and immunological properties led to the conclusion that all were functionally identical and all active fragments of the same precursor. The name lipocortin has been adopted and a human lipocortin has now been sequenced and cloned which shares many of the properties of both the early material and the glucocorticoid steroids.

The discovery of this protein explains why **puromycin**, an inhibitor of protein synthesis, will (by stopping the production of lipocortin) prevent the actions of **dexamethasone**. FFFFT

Plasma kinins include the nonapeptide bradykinin, which

1. is stored in cells as the decapeptide kallidin prior to release.
2. causes a slowing of the isolated heart.
3. stimulates sensory nerves to cause pain.
4. has actions all of which are inhibited by aspirin-like drugs.
5. is released in cutaneous inflammatory reactions.

Bradykinin (a nonapeptide; K9) is produced by the proteolytic enzyme, kallikrein, acting on a plasma α_2-globulin. This enzyme is usually present as a precursor in a variety of tissues and body fluids and is activated by trypsin, snake venoms or contact with foreign surfaces. Two other kinins exist (K10, lys-bradykinin or kallidin; and K11, met-lys-bradykinin) with properties similar to bradykinin; both can be converted to bradykinin. All have short half-lives (<30 s), inactivation being by plasma kininases.

Guinea-pig isolated ileum contracts on exposure to **bradykinin**, often after a latent period of several seconds (hence the name: *brady* = slow, *kinin* = movement). With some species (e.g. mouse) the isolated intestine first relaxes, then later contracts. **Bradykinin** causes a direct relaxant effect but it also releases substances like prostaglandins, whose spasmogenic effects later predominate. The complex effects of **bradykinin** on some other tissues may also be partly direct and partly indirect through the actions of secondarily released substances.

In addition to causing a direct vasodilatation and an increase in venular permeability to plasma proteins, **bradykinin** also stimulates sensory nerves. It therefore causes pain, an effect potentiated by prostaglandins, which themselves have little effect on sensory nerves. These three actions of **bradykinin** are responsible for the 'triple response', an acute inflammatory reaction in skin which can also be provoked by a variety of stimuli (allergies, exposure to heat, chemicals). The resemblance between the effects of **bradykinin** and these other stimuli as well as the fact that bradykinin is detected in inflamed tissues are among the reasons why it is thought to be a mediator of inflammation.

Receptors for **bradykinin** appear to exist in at least two forms. A few selective inhibitors are known, principally peptides. The synthesis of kinins can be blocked by the kallikrein inhibitor **aprotinin**. Also, aspirin-like drugs antagonize the bronchoconstrictor effects and curtail the vasodepressor responses of guinea-pigs to **bradykinin**. The antagonism presumably occurs because released prostaglandins are responsible and their biosynthesis is blocked by non-steroidal anti-inflammatory drugs such as **aspirin** or **ibuprofen**. This latter drug has become available as an over-the-counter remedy for inflammatory conditions as a result of many years of safe use on prescription. FFTFT.

MCQ 119

Polypeptides with actions on blood vessels include

1. bradykinin, whose breakdown is blocked by the same drugs which inhibit the synthesis of angiotensin II.
2. renin, a nonapeptide with vasoconstrictor effects found in the kidney.
3. vasoactive intestinal peptide and substance P, both of which are vasodilators.
4. angiotensin II and bradykinin, both of which are polypeptides formed in plasma.
5. antidiuretic hormone produced in the juxtaglomerular cells.

In addition to plasma kinins like bradykinin, other vasodilator peptides exist, for instance vasoactive intestinal peptide (VIP; 28 amino acids) and substance P (an undecapeptide). They both have a variety of other actions and are thought to be principally neurotransmitters or neuromodulators. Vasoconstrictor peptides also exist like vasopressin (alias antidiuretic hormone, a nonapeptide from the posterior pituitary) and angiotensin. There are interrelationships between angiotensin II and bradykinin as described below.

Like the precursor for bradykinin, that for angiotensin is a plasma α_2-globulin which is cleaved by the protease enzyme renin to an inactive decapeptide, angiotensin I. Renin is synthesized and released by juxtaglomerular cells in the kidney in response to

(a) decreased stretch of renal vascular receptors;
(b) decreased delivery of Na^+ and Cl^- to the macula densa;
(c) stimulation of β-adrenoceptors. Inhibition of renin release occurs with many vasoconstrictor substances.

The active octapeptide angiotensin II is formed from angiotensin I by the action of a peptidyl dipeptidase, called 'converting enzyme'. This enzyme is identical with the 'kininase II' which metabolizes bradykinin. In the lungs a reciprocal relationship occurs between these two peptides because a single enzyme is responsible for producing a powerful vasoconstrictor (angiotensin II) and inactivating a potent vasodilator (bradykinin). The half-life of angiotensin II is <60 s but its vasoconstrictor potency is high (about 50 times greater than noradrenaline). Part of its hypertensive effect is central, the peptide acting on the area postrema near the medulla oblongata to which it gains access through the poorly developed blood–brain barrier in that region. Angiotensin II also stimulates aldosterone secretion leading to Na^+ retention, which may contribute to the peptide's hypertensive effects. Antagonism of angiotensin is likely to lower the blood pressure. The most effective means of achieving blockade has been through inhibition of synthesis. Therefore drugs like **captopril** and **enalapril** (an ester which is hydrolysed in the plasma to an active metabolite), which are orally active inhibitors of 'converting enzyme', are used as antihypertensive drugs; a component of their action could result from the simultaneous preservation of bradykinin.

Other peptides with vasoconstrictor effects include neuropeptide-Y (also a putative CNS neuromodulator) and endothelin, one of several substances from endothelial cells which are thought to help regulate vascular tone.
TFTTF

5-Hydroxytryptamine

1. is stored in larger amounts in gut mucosa than in any other part of the mammalian body.
2. is a widely distributed CNS neurotransmitter with principally inhibitory effects.
3. causes relaxation of gut smooth muscle, for example rat stomach strip.
4. stimulates sensory nerves, causing pain or itching.
5. is considered an important mediator of acute inflammation in man.

5-Hydroxytryptamine (serotonin; 5-HT) is widely distributed in the mammalian body (e.g. CNS neurones, blood platelets and, principally, enterochromaffin cells of the gut). However, its physiological functions are a matter of debate and may vary between species. Undoubtedly it has neurotransmitter functions: 5-HT-containing nerves have cell bodies in the raphe nucleus, the pons and upper brainstem and their terminals are widespread; in most brain locations 5-HT has inhibitory effects associated with hyperpolarization.

On the gut, **5-HT** causes contraction but the sensitivity is greatly influenced by both the intestinal region and the species of animal from which the gut is derived. The rat is one of the most sensitive species and preparations like stomach fundus strip have been used for bioassay purposes. While 5-HT might serve as a local hormone, helping to control intestinal muscle tone, its role is unlikely to be crucial since antagonists are not notable in causing constipation. However, the excess of 5-HT produced by carcinoid tumours of enterochromaffin cells causes severe diarrhoea.

5-Hydroxytryptamine has pronounced effects on peripheral nerves and blood vessels. By stimulating sensory nerves, it causes itch or pain (as do autacoids like histamine and bradykinin). In rats and mice, oedema results from an increase in venular permeability to plasma proteins; 5-HT may contribute to local inflammatory reactions in these species since it is found in rodent mast cells in greater abundance than in other mammals. On vascular smooth muscle, 5-HT has complex actions which are probably determined by the subtype of 5-HT receptor that is activated. Most isolated blood vessels contract. However, *in vivo*, a fall in blood pressure may occur and complex multiphasic pressure changes probably result from a combination of effects of 5-HT on the vessels themselves, the heart, sensory nerves and on ganglionic transmission. TTFTF

MCQ 121

Receptors for 5-hydroxytryptamine

1. are classified according to their location in the body.
2. have been found on venular and arteriolar smooth muscle.
3. are termed 5-HT$_1$ if they are blocked by **ketanserin**.
4. of several subtypes have been isolated and cloned.
5. are involved in migraine.

5-Hydroxytryptamine (serotonin; 5-HT) is widely distributed in the mammalian body. Several types of cell (e.g. neurones, platelets) store 5-HT and binding sites for 5-HT have been found on a variety of cells both centrally and peripherally. These sites have been studied extensively in recent years. In the 1950s, 5-HT was postulated to act on two types of receptor, called M and D after **morphine** and **dibenamine**, both substances being required to block completely its spasmogenic actions on guinea-pig gut. Recent work has revealed that binding sites for 5-HT fall into three main types and several subtypes: 5-HT$_2$ and 5-HT$_3$, defined pharmacologically with selective antagonists; and 5-HT$_1$-like (further divided into 1A, 1B, 1C, 1D), characterized with selective agonists and, as yet, non-selective antagonists. However, as is found in other areas of pharmacology, *functional* receptors do not necessarily correlate with ligand binding sites in subcellular fragments.

The most common type on smooth muscle of arteries and veins is the 5-HT$_2$ receptor. This is classified on the basis of blockade by **ketanserin**, **ritanserin** or **cyproheptadine** and the failure of the substance **MDL-72222** (a selective 5-HT$_3$ antagonist) to cause blockade. Through stimulation of 5-HT$_2$ receptors, vasoconstriction occurs and the antihypertensive effects of **ketanserin** are explained partly on the basis of 5-HT antagonism and partly through its blocking action on vascular α_1-adrenoceptors. **Ketanserin** also counteracts platelet aggregation induced by 5-HT.

In some vessels, contraction appears to be mediated by 5-HT$_1$-like receptors, a selective *agonist* at which is the indole sulphonamide **GR-43175**. This substance has been used to investigate the possible roles of 5-HT in migraine and to test the conflicting vascular and neurogenic theories on the origin of migraine. **GR-43175** relieves or prevents all the symptoms of migraine while causing constriction of extracerebral cranial vessels, suggesting these may be the sites of pain production. However, it should be noted that several drugs used prophylactically, for example **methysergide** and **cyproheptadine**, are potent *blockers* at 5-HT$_2$ (and 5-HT$_{1c}$) sites; furthermore, 5-HT releasing drugs and a 5-HT$_{1c}$ agonist have been shown to trigger or exacerbate migraine attacks. The genesis of migraine may involve the activation of 5-HT neurones and, for example, 5-HT$_2$ receptors in the CNS, which leads to extracerebral vascular dilatation, thereby stimulating nociceptive afferent fibres in the vessel walls. Thus relief may be afforded by drug action at any of several sites, neuronal and/or vascular.

A greater understanding of proteins has resulted from the use of molecular biology techniques. For instance, fragments of DNA from one species can be inserted into bacterial cells. Clones of bacteria containing the new DNA will synthesize the corresponding protein in abundance, permitting its analysis and experimental use. Drug receptors are proteins and large quantities of some receptor molecules including several subtypes of 5-HT receptors have been produced by similar molecular biology techniques. FTFTT

The drug sodium cromoglycate

1. is not given by mouth to treat asthma because it is not absorbed from the gut.
2. is ineffective against exercise-induced asthma because of its selectivity for IgE-mediated reactions.
3. antagonizes the actions of several autacoids released from mast cells.
4. should be given just after the start of an asthmatic attack for optimal effect.
5. cannot reduce the pulmonary anaphylactic reactions caused in guinea-pigs by egg albumin.

Sodium cromoglycate (SCG) is a bis-cromone, structurally related to the alkaloid **khellin**. It was discovered during the early 1960s at a time when pharmacologists were developing animal models of human allergies mediated by reaginic antibodies. **Sodium cromoglycate** was shown to inhibit reagin-dependent cutaneous reactions in the rat. However, in the guinea-pig neither the allergic cutaneous reaction nor the lung reactions, which were mediated by other types of antibody, were inhibited by **SCG**.

Experimental models, like that in the rat, became acceptable when **SCG** was shown to be effective against human bronchial asthma. It also inhibited allergic release of autacoids from isolated human lung fragments. However, its specificity for reagin-mediated events is questionable, because it is known to combat exercise-induced asthma in which no immunological component is involved. Furthermore, experiments in dogs on reflex bronchoconstrictor responses show that **SCG** is capable, in therapeutic amounts, of inhibiting firing in some sensory nerves. Actions like these may contribute to its clinical effectiveness. **Sodium cromoglycate** is not a bronchodilator substance and it does not inhibit the effect of histamine or other mediators on smooth muscle.

Although soluble in water, **SCG** is very poorly absorbed from the gastrointestinal tract. Its routes of administration are, therefore, chosen to get the drug directly to its sites of action. For conjunctivitis there are eye-drops, for rhinitis a nasal spray, and for asthma the drug is more frequently given as a dry powder for inhalation from a Spinhaler, though a pressurized aerosol formulation is also available. Administration is prophylactic and few undesirable effects have been reported. Many patients fail to show improvement in objective spirometric tests, yet experience a subjective well-being while on **SCG**. they may be able to reduce the dosage of, or even eliminate, other drugs from their therapeutic regime. TFFFT

MCQ 123

Corticosteroids must be used with caution in asthmatic patients

1. because they may cause or aggravate peptic ulcers.
2. although **beclomethasone**, given by inhalation, is poorly absorbed and is less likely than most to cause systemic effects.
3. since by suppressing inflammatory reactions they may permit infections to go untreated until dangerous situations occur.
4. because they cause atrophy of the pituitary gland after several months use.
5. as they may give rise to osteoporosis by stimulating calcium excretion and accelerating protein breakdown.

When corticosteroids were introduced into clinical practice during the early 1950s, they were hailed as miracle drugs. However, they were soon used with caution because the incidence of undesirable effects was very high. Even synthetic steroids with minimal mineralocorticoid activity (**betamethasone, dexamethasone**) were potentially dangerous. They increased calcium excretion which, together with a tendency to break down protein, could lead to osteoporosis. They depressed production of lymphocytes and inhibited antibody formation (immunosuppressant). They suppressed corticotrophin (adrenocorticotrophic hormone) output from the pituitary gland, which caused decreased production of adrenal corticoids leading to atrophy of the adrenal cortex. They produced gastrointestinal upsets, and peptic ulcers were aggravated or sometimes induced.

Because of this pattern of effects, the steroids came to be used only as a treatment for refractory asthma or for status asthmaticus. In the early 1970s an aerosol form of **beclomethasone** was introduced for the management of asthma. This synthetic steroid, used previously in a formulation for topical application, is not absorbed from the gut and, therefore, an oral dose would be ineffective. Applied by aerosol it has antiasthmatic activity but too little is absorbed to affect adversely the pituitary–adrenal axis. **Beclomethasone** is now available in powder form for inhalation from a 'Rotahaler', frequently used by children. It is often prescribed for routine treatment instead of being reserved, like other steroids, for the management of intractable cases. Its most frequent unwanted effect is to permit oral growth of *Candida albicans* ('thrush'), which can be controlled by antifungal agents.

Asthmatic patients are often treated with more than one drug (e.g. aerosol steroid plus oral steroid or steroid plus bronchodilator). Clinical trials have been initiated with high-dose **beclomethasone** inhalations (up to 2 mg daily in divided doses instead of the more usual 0.3–0.5 mg). In many cases a reduction has been possible in the amount of oral steroids (e.g. **prednisolone**) given, thereby reducing the severity of unwanted effects. TTTFT

Sympathomimetic bronchodilator drugs which may be used in the management of allergic bronchial asthma

1. no longer include **isoprenaline** because of its lack of selectivity.
2. include **ephedrine**, which is active orally.
3. produce a lower incidence of cardiotoxicity the more selective they are for β_2-adrenoceptors.
4. will be ineffective if given prophylactically.
5. include the long-acting **salbutamol**, which is not biotransformed by catechol *O*-methyltransferase.

Both **adrenaline** (given s.c. or by inhalation) and **ephedrine** (an indirectly acting sympathomimetic drug, active orally and with a longer duration of action than **adrenaline**) have been used as bronchodilator drugs. Neither is used extensively nowadays because they both lack specificity. **Ephedrine** has pronounced CNS effects and **adrenaline** stimulates cardiac β_1-adrenoceptors as well as α-adrenoceptors.

Isoprenaline largely replaced these drugs in the 1950s and was later formulated in a convenient metered-dose aerosol. In the mid-1960s an increase in the mortality rate in European asthmatics was correlated with an increased use of **isoprenaline** aerosols, especially in a high-dosage formulation. It was concluded that many sudden deaths were caused by an excess of **isoprenaline** stimulating cardiac β_1-adrenoceptors and inducing fatal dysrhythmias (particularly likely during hypoxia). There is evidence that the inhaled fluorocarbon propellants additionally sensitized the myocardium to sympathetic stimulation.

Research which led to the subdivision in the classification of β-adreno-ceptors also led to the development of drugs selective for the subgroups and **salbutamol** appeared as the prototype β_2-adrenoceptor agonist. Given by aerosol or by mouth (its non-catechol structure preserving the drug from attack by catechol *O*-methyltransferase), the drug has little action on the heart in bronchodilator doses, but overdose causes the typical inotropic and chronotropic response associated with β_1-adrenoceptor stimulation. Several other drugs also selective for β_2-adrenoceptors have been developed (e.g. **terbutaline**, **rimiterol**, **fenoterol**).

These drugs are generally recommended for use after an asthmatic attack has begun (i.e. to be employed for their bronchodilator activity). However, they also inhibit the release of autacoids from mast cells (possibly through a β-adrenoceptor-linked adenylate cyclase). For this reason it has been recommended that **salbutamol** may be used prophylactically by asthma sufferers. FTTFT

MCQ 125

Allergic bronchial asthma may be treated with

1. sympathomimetic drugs which selectively block the β_2-adrenoceptors of airway smooth muscle.
2. antihistamine drugs blocking H_2-receptors.
3. atropinic drugs, like **ipratropium**, which is administered by inhalation.
4. corticosteroids, like **prednisolone**, which is active when taken by mouth.
5. **aspirin**, which inhibits the biosynthesis of the bronchoconstrictor prostaglandin E_2.

Bronchial asthma is characterized by breathlessness and wheezing and there is an increased responsiveness of airway smooth muscle to a variety of stimuli. Commonly the cause is allergic and then the immunological mediator is usually reaginic antibody (IgE).

Drugs used in this condition may be classified in four groups.

Bronchodilators act as functional antagonists to bronchoconstrictor autacoids. They include sympathomimetic drugs which stimulate the β_2-adrenoceptors in the airway smooth muscle (e.g. **salbutamol, isoprenaline**) and methylxanthines which may act either through inhibition of the enzyme phosphodiesterase or by blocking adenosine receptors (e.g. **theophylline**).

The second group consists of the *pharmacological antagonists* of histamine, which seems of little importance in bronchial asthma but is a major autacoid in hay fever. Its effects on the airways are relieved by H_1-receptor blockers (e.g. **mepyramine**). Increased vagal efferent activity often accompanies inhalation of allergenic substances and, together with an increased sensitivity to acetylcholine, this explains why muscarinic receptor blockers are sometimes useful (e.g. **ipratropium bromide**).

Inhibitors of mediator release constitute a third group, exemplified by **sodium cromoglycate**, which reduces the release from mast cells of autacoids like histamine and eicosanoids. It is ineffective when asthmatic attacks have begun but is given prophylactically. Interestingly, the bronchodilator drugs have been shown in animal models also to inhibit mediator release (the mast cell is stabilized when its β-adrenoceptors are stimulated or when phosphodiesterase is blocked, both of which raise cyclic AMP levels). However, the bronchodilators tend to be used clinically when respiratory distress is experienced, too late to block the output of mediators.

Anti-inflammatory drugs make up the last group. The non-steroidal drugs are not effective (indeed, **aspirin** may cause asthmatic attacks in sensitive patients). Corticosteroids (like **prednisolone**) are useful, however; they have been shown to decrease arachidonic acid production and so reduce production of all eicosanoids. FFTTF

Central Nervous System

MCQ 126

Pharmacological receptors in the CNS

1. are predominantly either cholinoceptors or adrenoceptors.
2. which are non-functional can be distinguished from functional receptors by ligand binding studies.
3. are unevenly distributed through the brain.
4. are present in numbers which may decrease gradually with age but otherwise remain relatively constant.
5. belong to at least 40 different types.

Some 30 or more chemical substances have been postulated as possible neurotransmitters or neuromodulators in the CNS. Many act at more than one type of receptor (e.g. adrenaline on α_1-, α_2- and β_1-adrenoceptors) and 40 is an underestimate of the number of different receptor types in the CNS.

Ligand binding studies *in vitro* have demonstrated a great number of binding sites, some of which have the affinity and specificity characteristic of receptors. Other binding sites may be associated with transporter systems (e.g. the 5-hydroxytryptamine (5-HT) uptake system). It must be remembered that just because a binding site has the characteristics of a receptor it is not necessarily a *functional* receptor able to modify CNS activity; more importantly it does not have to be associated with any behavioural or physiological function. In particular brain regions, some receptors may be present at higher density (e.g. adrenoceptors in the hypothalamus; cholinoceptors in the forebrain) but in the brain as a whole these two receptor sites form only a small proportion of the total receptor population. Noradrenaline, dopamine, 5-HT, acetylcholine, histamine, amino acids (glutamine, γ-aminobutyric acid, glycine) and a host of neuropeptides are known to be present in the CNS, synthesized and stored locally, unevenly distributed, released during neuronal activity and quickly removed; all characteristics expected of a neurotransmitter. In only a small number of cases has a link been established between a particular transmitter and a specific function (e.g. dopamine in movement control; noradrenaline in mood and central control of blood pressure). Even in these examples a full understanding of the pathways involved has not been achieved.

The number of receptors in the CNS can change due to ageing or to disease processes and can also be modified by drugs. Chronic treatment with drugs can cause up-regulation (increases) or down-regulation (decreases) in receptor numbers (e.g. antidepressants up-regulate β-adrenoceptors). The mechanisms involved in these processes are not fully understood but are likely to be important as many drugs acting on the CNS produce some of their effects only after a delay of several days or weeks, during which time receptor regulation may take place (e.g. antipsychotic agents). FFTFT

An example of a CNS transmitter and the receptor type with which it interacts is

1. histamine with H₃-receptors.
2. pro-dynorphin with mu opioid receptors.
3. β-endorphin with kappa opioid receptors.
4. Leu-enkephalin with kappa opioid receptors.
5. substance P with P₁-receptors.

The original concept of 'neurotransmitter' encompassed a substance released from a neurone which produced a fast and transient effect on the excitability of an adjacent cell. The concept has been modified now that it is appreciated that substances may:

(a) affect the neurone from which they were released;
(b) produce effects which are slow in onset or of long (hours) duration;
(c) act diffusely at points distant from their release;
(d) affect not only excitability but also, for example, transmitter synthesis or the number of receptors.

Some authors use the terms neuromodulator or neuroregulator to cover such substances but there is no generally agreed definition of these terms.

Histamine is synthesized and stored in some CNS neurones and is found more diffusely distributed throughout the CNS in mast cells. **Histamine** can stimulate a histamine-sensitive adenylate cyclase and, given microiontophoretically, can cause both excitatory (H_1-mediated) and inhibitory (H_2-mediated) effects on neuronal firing. A histamine receptor (H_3) has been identified on histaminergic neurones, functioning as an autoreceptor controlling histamine release through a negative feedback mechanism (analogous to the presynaptic α_2-adrenoceptor of noradrenergic nerves). A major functional role for histamine in the CNS seems unlikely in view of the minor CNS effects (other than sedation) of both H_1- and H_2-receptor blockers such as **mepyramine** and **ranitidine** respectively.

Several opioid receptors have been characterized and are designated mu, delta, kappa and sigma. Stimulation is associated with particular effects: mu – analgesia at supraspinal levels, respiratory depression, euphoria and physical dependence; kappa – analgesia at spinal levels, sedation, pupillary constriction; sigma – dysphoria and hallucinations; delta – inhibition of transmitter release from neurones. Many peptide transmitters (neuro-peptides) are known to stimulate these opioid receptors. The neuropeptides are derived from large protein molecules (about 250 residues) such as pro-opiomelanocortin (yielding β-endorphin; mu, delta and kappa receptors), pro-enkephalin (leu- and met-enkephalin; mu and delta receptors) and pro-dynorphin (dynorphin; mu and kappa receptors).

Substance P is an undecapeptide (11 amino acids), concentrated in neurones of the dorsal roots of the spinal cord both in the periphery (where release, in the triple response for example, causes vasodilatation and extravasation of fluid) and in primary afferents in the dorsal horn (where it may have a nociceptive transmitter role). Other neuropeptides which

continued on next page 157

occur in different areas of the dorsal horn and may also have transmitter roles include vasoactive intestinal peptide (VIP), somatostatin and cholecystokinin C-terminal octapeptide (CCK-8).

The term P_1-receptors refers to a type of purine receptor on which adenosine is more potent than ATP and which is blocked by **theophylline**. Adenosine triphosphate is more potent than adenosine at P_2-receptors. Adenosine and ATP may have roles as transmitters and/or co-transmitters in both the CNS and the periphery, as also may many of the peptides listed above. TFTFF

An example of a CNS transmitter and the receptor type with which it interacts is

1. γ-aminobutyric acid with GABA$_A$- and GABA$_B$-receptors.
2. glycine with receptors blocked by **strychnine**.
3. **N-methyl-D-aspartate** with L-glutamate receptors.
4. γ-aminobutyric acid with receptors blocked by **bicucculline**.
5. L-glutamate with **quisqualate** receptors.

γ-Aminobutyric acid (GABA) is formed from glutamate by glutamic acid decarboxylase and is found in all brain areas but is particularly concentrated in the nigrostriatal region. It is destroyed by GABA transaminase (located in mitochondria) but, as with noradrenaline, reuptake and diffusion are mainly responsible for removing GABA from the synapse. GABA$_A$-receptors are stimulated by GABA and **muscimol**, are located primarily postsynaptically and increase the chloride conductance of cells. This leads to hyper-polarization of the cell and an inhibition of firing; hence the general classification of GABA as an inhibitory transmitter.

Competitive (**bicucculline**) and non-competitive (**picrotoxin**) blockers of these receptors, not surprisingly, have CNS stimulant and proconvulsant actions. The interaction of GABA with these receptors is potentiated by benzodiazepines, which probably bind to discrete benzodiazepine receptors. These, like the GABA receptors, are associated with a chloride channel. The binding sites for benzodiazepines in the brain closely parallel the distribution of GABA$_A$-receptors. Benzodiazepine receptors do not operate the chloride channel but increase the affinity of GABA$_A$-receptors for GABA and so enhance the action of GABA and produce sedative and anticonvulsant effects.

GABA$_B$-receptors are primarily located presynaptically, where they inhibit release of transmitters possibly by reducing influx of calcium ions which is essential for exocytosis. GABA$_B$-receptors are stimulated by GABA, **baclofen** and **2-hydroxysaclofen**.

Glycine is found in high concentrations in the grey matter of the cord, where it produces hyperpolarization and hence inhibition. Its action is blocked by **strychnine** and its release is inhibited by **tetanus toxin**; both of these materials cause convulsions.

The naturally occurring amino acids L-aspartate and L-glutamate have excitatory actions on the CNS. The latter compound is widely and fairly evenly distributed within the CNS but this probably reflects a metabolic role since it is involved in both carbohydrate and nitrogen metabolism. The most compelling evidence for a transmitter role for L-glutamate is in the hippo-campus and the olfactory tract, where it increases conductance of sodium and of other cations. Three distinct receptor subtypes for these amino acids are now recognized, named after the three agonists which show some selectivity: **N-methyl-D-aspartate** (NMDA), **quisqualate** and **kainate**. The first of these, NMDA, is not a naturally occurring substance (note its D-configuration); it has been intensively studied and mimics closely many of the actions of glutamate. A variety of **NMDA** antagonists are known, acting competitively or non-competitively and the search continues for others because of their clinical potential to treat conditions like epilepsy, stroke, anxiety and schizophrenia. TTFTT

MCQ 129

The central nervous system depressant

1. **chloral hydrate** is used as a hypnotic principally in the young and the elderly.
2. effect of the antihistamine **diphenhydramine** is, for all practical purposes, non-existent.
3. **urethane** is a useful hypnotic in man.
4. **glutethimide** may reduce motion sickness.
5. **methaqualone** is unlikely to produce dependence.

Chloral hydrate is a moderately strong hypnotic and is used particularly in children and in the elderly though its disagreeable taste makes it unpleasant to take. It potentiates **ethanol** strongly and induces microsomal enzymes. It has a wider safety margin than the barbiturates. It is a pro-drug, being biotransformed to trichloroethanol, which is the active material causing the hypnotic effect.

Diphenhydramine, like most antihistamines acting at H_1-receptors, is a CNS depressant and therefore causes drowsiness whenever it is used to treat allergies or motion sickness. This mild hypnotic action is effective in children (except in the children of one of the authors on long flights!) and is accompanied by few unpleasant effects. The drug has a wide safety margin.

Urethane (ethyl carbamate) is never used as a hypnotic in man because in large doses it depresses the bone marrow and because it is associated with the development of cancer. For this reason it must be handled with care in laboratories. However, it may be given i.p. or i.v. as a 'non-recovery anaesthetic' in experimental animals, where its effects last for several hours. Lacking aromatic rings, **urethane** is of simple chemical structure and interferes little with chemical assays of body fluid constituents. It raises levels of catecholamines by stimulating their release, an effect which must be borne in mind when choosing an anaesthetic for a particular series of experiments.

Glutethimide is similar in effect to 'medium-duration' barbiturates. It shares many of their disadvantages like tolerance, dependence, disturbances of rapid-eye movement (REM) sleep and a small safety margin. However, it has atropinic actions, which cause dry mouth, blurred vision and reduced gastrointestinal motility. The atropinic effect may account for its antimotion sickness action since many drugs used for this purpose share that property.

Methaqualone is an effective hypnotic but disturbs REM sleep, produces tolerance and dependence and is, in addition, a cough suppressant. Dependence is especially likely to occur when it is combined with **diphenhydramine** (Mandrax; street name 'Mandies'), the combination being a drug of abuse.

Chloral hydrate, **diphenhydramine** and, much less frequently, **glutethimide**, all find a use as hypnotic agents in particular circumstances. In terms of general hypnotic–sedative use, however, nearly all these drugs have been superseded by the benzodiazepines. TFFTF

Hypnotic or sedative drugs may be used

1. to calm an anxious patient.
2. to induce sleep in a patient suffering from pain.
3. as primary therapy in a psychotic patient.
4. safely in combination with **ethanol**.
5. for prolonged periods without harmful effects.

Hypnotics are used to induce or maintain sleep, while sedatives will calm an anxious patient without producing sleep (although sleep will occur if the agent is given in a large enough dose at a suitable time and in an environment conducive to sleep). In many cases hypnotic drugs given in small doses will produce sedation. However, not all sedative drugs can be used as hypnotics since the necessarily increased dose may cause unacceptable side-effects.

Simple sedatives were once commonly used to treat anxiety but have largely been replaced by the minor tranquillizers (e.g. **diazepam**), which have sedative properties in addition to their anxiolytic action. Some other benzodiazepines (e.g. **nitrazepam, flurazepam**) which produce greater sedative or hypnotic effects in relation to their other actions, are marketed specifically as hypnotics. The benzodiazepines exert their effects through a binding site (benzodiazepine receptor) close to chloride channels on neuronal membranes. They do not directly affect chloride conductance, but increase the affinity of a neighbouring receptor, the $GABA_A$ receptor, for γ-aminobutyric acid (GABA) whose actions to increase chloride entry are thus enhanced. Therefore benzodiazepines have inhibitory actions by facilitating the effects of GABA. Similar enhancement might be expected from drugs which raise synaptic GABA concentrations, for example, by blocking autoinhibitory $GABA_B$ presynaptic receptors found on terminals of neurones which release GABA. **Baclofen** is a $GABA_B$ blocker and has been used to treat spastic conditions because of its muscle relaxing effects. Newer, alternative drugs may have useful sedative/hypnotic actions.

All sedative or hypnotic drugs are at least additive with **ethanol** and in some cases (e.g. with barbiturates) there is considerable potentiation. Generally, patients must be warned to avoid combinations of these drugs with alcoholic drinks.

The sensation of pain is increased by hypnotics and patients suffering pain will rarely be able to sleep unless massive doses are given or analgesics are employed as well. Hypnotics and sedatives do not have antipsychotic effects (unlike neuroleptic drugs). However, sleep disorders occurring during adequate antipsychotic therapy may be treated with hypnotics.

Prolonged therapy with hypnotics or sedatives is to be avoided as there is considerable evidence that in some patients cumulation, tolerance, dependence and other harmful effects may occur. TFFFF

MCQ 131

Ethanol

1. is biotransformed to methanal (formaldehyde).
2. biotransformation in the liver involves aldehyde dehydrogenase.
3. is a CNS stimulant.
4. can be used to treat **methanol** poisoning.
5. can produce tolerance.

About 98% of ingested **ethanol** is biotransformed by the hepatic enzyme alcohol dehydrogenase to ethanal (acetaldehyde) and then by aldehyde dehydrogenase to ethanoic (acetic) acid, which is utilized in the Krebs' cycle. It thus forms a ready supply of energy, liberating some 30 kJ per gram. The toxic products methanal (formaldehyde) and methanoic (formic) acid are the counterpart metabolites of **methanol**, which is added to industrial alcohols (e.g. methylated spirits, surgical spirit) to make them unfit for drinking. Thus Excise Duty, which is payable on all potable spirit, is not applicable. Drinking these spirits (or the inadvertent consumption of **methanol**) leads to blindness (a selective effect of methanal on the retina) and severe acidosis because methanoic acid is a very strong acid.

Since both of these alcohols are biotransformed by the same enzymes, **ethanol** can be administered to delay the biotransformation of **methanol**. The delay permits the body more time to excrete **methanol** (through the lungs and urine) and to cope with the toxic metabolites formed.

In spite of an apparent CNS stimulation in social use, **ethanol** has primarily central depressant actions. It first depresses inhibitory centres, thereby seeming to cause excitation. Fine judgement is impaired early though the imbiber is usually unaware of this (the driving problem!). Vasodilatation is produced in skin vessels: hence the correct belief that it is bad to take **alcohol** *before* being exposed to cold (increased heat loss) though good *after* exposure (vasodilatation giving a feeling of warmth). Larger doses of **alcohol** lead to coma and death.

Tolerance to **ethanol** is marked and dependence is becoming an increasing problem in society generally. Among the other undesirable effects of **ethanol**, especially in chronic use, are gastritis, loss of appetite (and hence nutritional deficiencies), cirrhosis of the liver and psychoses. FTFTT

In anaesthetic practice, the

1. depth of anaesthesia at equilibrium with gaseous agents will be increased if carbon dioxide is included in the inspired gas mixture.
2. rate of onset of gaseous anaesthesia will be faster if carbon dioxide is included in the inspired gas mixture.
3. use of narcotic analgesics will delay recovey from general anaesthesia.
4. anaesthetics **halothane** and **enflurane** sensitize the heart to the action of catecholamines.
5. anaesthetic **fluroxine** will potentiate the effects of **pancuronium**.

Inclusion of carbon dioxide in the inspired gas mixture will activate reflexes which increase the rate and depth of breathing. This will improve alveolar ventilation and speed the exchange of gas from which the anaesthetic has been absorbed with fresh, anaesthetic-containing gas. The rate of uptake of the anaesthetic into the bloodstream will, therefore, be increased and onset of anaesthesia will be faster. Equilibrium will occur more quickly, but the *depth* of anaesthesia *at equilibrium* will not be altered. It should be noted that, with some anaesthetics, true equilibrium takes many hours to be established and is rarely achieved in typical surgical cases.

Narcotic analgesics cause sedation (CNS depression), which will add to the depressant effect of the anaesthetic. More importantly, however, they depress respiration and therefore impede the clearance of anaesthetic from the lungs, delaying recovery.

Most of the halogenated anaesthetics sensitize the myocardium to the action of catecholamines, although the extent varies between drugs and is greater with **enflurane** than with **halothane**. Before and during anaesthesia, stress and anxiety greatly increase plasma catecholamine levels; cardiac dysrhythmias may result from these high levels especially if the myocardium has been sensitized to their action. Careful premedication with sedatives or tranquillizers and an explanatory visit from the anaesthetist before the operation can greatly reduce anxiety and consequently the risk associated with this effect.

In modern anaesthetic practice, anaesthesia is kept light and supplemented by other drugs (e.g. neuromuscular blockers like **tubocurarine, pancuronium, atracurium**). Most of the halogenated hydrocarbons potentiate the effect of neuromuscular blockers and the dose of the latter drugs must be reduced accordingly. Most of the neuromuscular blockers are of relatively short duration (30 min) but, if necessary, the effect of competitive blockers can be reversed at the end of the operation by an anticholinesterase agent (e.g. **neostigmine**). If this is done, care must be taken to ensure that the anticholinesterase effect will outlast the neuromuscular blockade or paralysis may return while the patient is still recovering. FTTTT

MCQ 133

General anaesthesia

1. may be produced by some steroids.
2. can be achieved by inhalation of **methohexitone**.
3. with **ketamine** may be more satisfactory in adults if **droperidol** is given preoperatively.
4. induced by **urethane** can be used for tonsillectomy in children.
5. with **thiopentone** would be contraindicated in a patient with acute intermittent porphyria.

The term 'steroid' merely describes a substance having four fused rings (cyclopentanoperhydrophenanthrene) in its chemical nucleus. Some compounds, **althesin** for example, are steroidal in nature but show none of the actions associated with the steroidal hormones. **Althesin** was a short-acting anaesthetic which produced little disturbance of blood pressure or respiration when given i.v. However, an increasing number of reports concerning severe allergic reactions has led to its withdrawal from clinical use.

Methohexitone and **thiopentone** also have a short duration (15–20 min) and fast onset (15 s) but are barbiturates and thus show most of the properties of this group. They are administered i.v. (as the sodium salts) and are alkaline. The highly caustic injections must be given with care so that none of the solution will escape the vein, or tissue damage will result. With barbiturates, respiration is depressed and laryngospasm may be produced. Liver microsomal enzymes are induced, including aminolaevulinic acid synthetase, which controls the rate of porphyrin synthesis. In normal patients this is of little consequence, but in patients with a defect in porphyrin breakdown (acute intermittent porphyria for example) an acute attack may be precipitated (severe abdominal pain, gastrointestinal disturbances, severe impairment of autonomic and motor nerve function, death).

Another short-acting i.v. anaesthetic is **etomidate**. The cardiovascular and respiratory systems are not usually depressed during the 5 min or so that the patient is unconscious. Involuntary muscle movements may occur which can be suppressed by drugs like **diazepam**.

Ketamine (given i.v. or i.m.) produces 'dissociative anaesthesia' of fast onset and short duration. The cardiovascular and respiratory systems are not depressed. The frightening hallucinations which are experienced by some adults during recovery from **ketamine** anaesthesia are minimized by pretreatment with **droperidol** (a butyrophenone major tranquillizer). These hallucinations occur much less frequently in children, in whom **ketamine** is often used for painful procedures, such as changing burn dressings.

Urethane (and **chloralose**) are long-lasting general anaesthetics used only in animals. **Urethane** should be handled with caution since it is associated with the development of cancer. TFTFT

In comparison with nitrous oxide, halothane

1. is more potent.
2. produces a greater analgesic effect.
3. is more soluble in blood.
4. produces a faster induction of anaesthesia.
5. is more likely to reduce blood pressure.

Halothane ($CF_3.CHClBr$) and **nitrous oxide** (N_2O) are widely used anaesthetics, though **nitrous oxide** is rarely used alone for anything but minor surgery. The two agents are often combined since their properties complement each other. **Halothane** is a volatile liquid (b.p. 50 °C) but **nitrous oxide** is a colourless gas at room temperature, stored under pressure as a liquid in cylinders (coloured blue).

The potency of a general anaesthetic is measured as the minimum alveolar concentration required to produce a given depth of anaesthesia. On this basis, **halothane** is over 100 times more potent than **nitrous oxide**. In practice, 0.5-1% **halothane** is used to maintain anaesthesia, while 80% **nitrous oxide** is still insufficient to produce full anaesthesia in some patients. Because such a high concentration of **nitrous oxide** is necessary, only 20% (atmospheric) oxygen can be inhaled in a mixture and there is a risk of hypoxia.

The blood–gas partition coefficient (solubility in blood) of **halothane** is 2.4 and of **nitrous oxide** 0.47, reflecting the greater solubility of **halothane** in blood. A large amount of **halothane** must be transported into the body to raise its partial pressure in the blood and this takes time. The rate of onset of anaesthesia with **nitrous oxide** is fast, while that of **halothane** is slow. To try to minimize this disadvantage, an initially high concentration of **halothane** (2-3%) is often administered to induce anaesthesia. Recovery from anaesthesia is also determined partially by solubility of the agent in the blood and is therefore very fast with **nitrous oxide**.

Nitrous oxide has excellent analgesic properties, while **halothane** is poor in this respect. This may seem irrelevant since the patient is unconscious, but there are still autonomic responses to pain and the stability of the cardiovascular system is often used to judge the state of a patient. **Nitrous oxide** is used at non-anaesthetic concentrations for its analgesic properties (**Entonox**: 50 : 50 nitrous oxide–oxygen) in childbirth and is carried in accident and emergency vehicles. A high oxygen tension and relief from pain is thus provided without the risk of respiratory depression seen with narcotic analgesics.

Halothane depresses respiration but the response to carbon dioxide remains during light anaesthesia. The myocardium is also depressed and blood pressure falls. **Nitrous oxide** is relatively free from effects on blood pressure and respiration. TFTFT

MCQ 135

In comparison with halothane *the general anaesthetic* isoflurane *is*

1. more potent.
2. more expensive.
3. more soluble in blood.
4. metabolized to a greater extent in man.
5. more likely to induce cardiac dysrhythmias.

Isoflurane ($CF_3.CHCl.O.CHF_2$) and **halothane** ($CF_3.CHClBr$) are both halogenated anaesthetics but **isoflurane**, like **enflurane** ($CHFCl.CF_2.O.CHF_2$) and **methoxyflurane** ($CHCl_2.CF_2.O.CH_3$), has an ether link which modifies the anaesthetic properties. **Isoflurane** is a low boiling liquid (b.p. 48.5 °C; **halothane** 50.2 °C) which is generally stable and non-reactive but has a somewhat more pungent odour than **halothane** and this can lead to breath-holding if high concentrations are used during induction.

The potency of volatile general anaesthetics can be measured as the minimum alveolar concentration (MAC) necessary to maintain general anaesthesia. This is not a fixed value but depends on the characteristics (e.g. age) of the subjects in which it is determined and the conditions of the measurement. Mixed with oxygen alone, the MAC for **isoflurane** is about 1.3% (**halothane** 0.75%). Using a gas mixture containing 70% **nitrous oxide**, the MAC for **isoflurane** is about 0.56% while that for **halothane** is about 0.29%, again illustrating the greater potency of **halothane** and also demonstrating the dependence of the MAC on the conditions of the determination.

Solubility of a volatile anaesthetic in blood is measured by the blood–gas partition coefficient (1.4 and 2.3 for **isoflurane** and **halothane** respectively). The greater the value, the more soluble the agent and the greater the quantity which has to be transported into the blood from the lungs. This takes time and, generally, the more soluble the agent, the slower the induction of anaesthesia unless special procedures are adopted, for example using a high induction concentration of a soluble agent to ensure that a large quantity of anaesthetic is driven into the blood in a short time, so speeding induction.

It is well established that **halothane** can cause liver damage; this may appear as jaundice (up to 20% of patients) or as a severe and sometimes fatal massive liver necrosis (perhaps 1 in 100 000). It is thought that reactive metabolites, formed in the liver, may play a role in this problem along with an immunological component. About 15% of **halothane** may eventually be biotransformed compared with only about 0.2% of **isoflurane**. Therefore the risk of liver damage would appear to be reduced.

The risk of cardiac dysrhythmias, especially in stressed patients where circulating catecholamine levels are high, is increased by the ability of **halothane** to sensitize the heart to the dysrhythmic action of catecholamines. **Isoflurane** shares this action with **halothane** but to a markedly lesser extent.

The cost of the drugs may be considered irrelevant but in a cash-limited hospital budget any reduced risk from the use of **isoflurane** must be balanced against its costs; **isoflurane** is about 10 times more expensive than **halothane**. FTFFF

Some barbiturates have one principal clinical use such as

1. **methohexitone** for general anaesthesia.
2. **thiopentone** as a sedative.
3. **pentobarbitone** as a hypnotic.
4. **phenobarbitone** in the treatment of epilepsy.
5. **amylobarbitone** as a short-acting sedative.

All barbiturates possess a similar, wide spectrum of biological actions and tend to differ only quantitatively. Differences in potency, duration and latency of action largely dictate their individual therapeutic uses. Variations in distribution, biotransformation and excretion of the barbiturates are responsible for these differences.

Methohexitone and **thiopentone** are both termed 'ultra-short-acting' barbiturates and are given i.v. This requires care as the alkaline solutions are very caustic and will damage tissues if any escapes the vein. These drugs produce general anaesthesia within 15 s and this action is terminated after about 15–20 min by redistribution of the drug. The brain initially receives a large proportion of the injected dose since it is well perfused with blood. Redistribution occurs to other body tissues which are less well perfused and therefore take up the drug more slowly.

Pentobarbitone lasts 3 h after oral administration and is used as a hypnotic, as is **amylobarbitone**, which lasts 6–8 h. Both drugs may be used as general anaesthetics in laboratory mammals.

Phenobarbitone has marked antiepileptic properties and is very long-lasting. The use of barbiturates in general anaesthesia and against epilepsy is still perfectly justifiable, but their use as hypnotics or sedatives for longer than 2–3 days is not and they have been replaced by safer drugs (e.g. **diazepam**). The advantages of this substitution are apparent from the data on poisoning in the UK. About 20 years ago barbiturates were involved in 70% of all fatal poisonings; by 1982 the figure was 18% and by 1986 it had fallen even further to around 7%. It should not be inferred that barbiturates were the cause of death in every case nor that their replacements are absolutely safe. TFTTF

MCQ 137

Barbiturates may

1. reduce the time spent in rapid-eyeball-movement sleep.
2. produce useful analgesia.
3. induce hepatic microsomal enzymes.
4. depress respiration.
5. be eliminated faster in an acid urine.

It is now appreciated that the nature of sleep is probably more important than its duration and several distinct types or phases of sleep have been identified. Many hypnotic drugs, barbiturates in particular, disturb the pattern and timing of the different types of sleep. Rapid-eye movement (REM) sleep especially is reduced by barbiturates and the period of sleep, though extended, is not refreshing. On withdrawal of the barbiturate, a period of excessive REM sleep is experienced (rebound 'remming'). Other disadvantages of barbiturates, when used clinically as hypnotics, are:

(a) induction of hepatic enzymes (thus giving rise to drug interactions);
(b) dependence and automatism;
(c) risk of fatal overdose;
(d) potentiation of the effects of **ethanol**;
(e) cumulation;
(f) hangover;
(g) impairment of skills and fine judgement for as long as 24 h after a dose is administered.

For all these reasons newer hypnotics are preferred, though it should not be thought that the newer drugs are trouble-free.

Should overdose occur, attempts should be made to minimize further absorption of the barbiturate (stomach wash). Removal of absorbed drug is encouraged by haemodialysis or peritoneal dialysis in extreme cases, but more usually by establishing an alkaline diuresis (**frusemide** and **sodium bicarbonate**). In an alkaline urine, more of the barbiturate (weak acid) exists in the ionized form and, therefore, less will be reabsorbed into the bloodstream from the lumen of the kidney tubule. More is thus excreted. Respiration, cardiovascular function, nutrition and blood chemistry may require support. The patient may be comatose so care must be taken to avoid hypostatic pneumonia. Central nervous system stimulants such as **bemegride** were once used to counteract the depressant action of the barbiturates but nowadays most authorities agree that the routine use of stimulants does not improve the clinical outcome. TFTTF

The benzodiazepine

1. group of drugs block $GABA_B$-receptors in the CNS.
2. **diazepam** has a longer duration of action than **temazepam**.
3. **midazolam** is used primarily to treat epilepsy.
4. **clonazepam** is used primarily as a hypnotic.
5. group of drugs interacts with **cimetidine**, which induces liver enzymes and therefore reduces benzodiazepine actions.

γ-Aminobutyric acid (GABA) receptors, $GABA_A$ not $GABA_B$, are closely associated with the chloride ion channel, which opens when these receptors are activated by GABA itself or other $GABA_A$ agonists (**muscimol**). Chloride ions flow into the cell, cause hyperpolarization and inhibit cell firing. Hence the classification of GABA as an inhibitory transmitter. Benzodiazepine binding sites are associated with the chloride channel–GABA–receptor complex and an agonist action at the benzodiazepine receptor will enhance the binding of GABA to its receptor and therefore intensify the actions of GABA. Thus benzodiazepines like **diazepam** have inhibitory actions (sleep promotion, anticonvulsant, antianxiety, centrally mediated muscle relaxation, amnesia). All agonists at benzodiazepine receptors share these actions though particular agents may be marketed as if they possessed only one of these effects (e.g. **nitrazepam** for sleep). Benzodiazepine partial agonists show a similar spectrum of action.

Benzodiazepine antagonists (**flumazenil**) will block the binding of benzodiazepine agonists or partial agonists and could therefore be used in the treatment of overdose. Compounds are known which will bind to the benzodiazepine receptor and cause a *decrease* in the binding of GABA to $GABA_A$-receptors. Since the actions of GABA are consequently reduced, these drugs are anxiogenic and proconvulsant and are known as inverse agonists.

Major differences exist in the pharmacokinetics of benzodiazepines (of which there are at least 15 on the market) and often determine their patterns of clinical use. **Temazepam** and **triazolam** are short-acting and are used primarily as hypnotics (half-life $(t_{1/2})$ about 6 and 3 h respectively; no hangover on waking); **triazolam** may take longer to be absorbed than **temazepam** and therefore may work less quickly. **Diazepam** $(t_{1/2}$ about 40 h) is used as an antianxiety agent, where the more prolonged action makes for a smooth maintenance of effect. Many benzodiazepines are biotransformed through pathways that are inhibited by **cimetidine**, which prolongs and intensifies their action. However, biotransformation may produce an active product with a longer duration of action than the parent (e.g. **diazepam** to **desmethyldiazepam**; $t_{1/2}$ about 60 h). This contributes to one of the several problems associated with prolonged benzodiazepine therapy: cumulation of parent drug or active metabolite in the body. This occurs especially in the elderly and may also contribute to the prolonged (>36 h) sedation, drowsiness and impairment of skills produced by some benzodiazepines.

continued on next page 169

Tolerance and dependence develop on prolonged use; 'coming off tranx' can be very difficult and those involved may benefit from membership of support groups formed for mutual help. Therapy should always involve low doses given for short periods. The tolerance makes benzodiazepines generally less than satisfactory as anticonvulsants (except in status epilepticus, where tolerance development is not relevant) though tolerance to **clonazepam** and **clobazam** may develop more slowly, which is why these agents are used in preference to others when a chronic antiepileptic effect is required.

Midazolam is more water-soluble than other benzodiazepines and can be given i.v. to provide sedation for procedures like gastroscopy. **Diazepam** can also be given i.v. either as an emulsion or in a special solvent, although some pain and irritation of the vein may be produced. FTFFF

The benzodiazepine nitrazepam

1. is superior to **midazolam** as an anxiolytic.
2. shows anticonvulsant and muscle relaxant activity.
3. shows sedative–hypnotic and anxiolytic activity.
4. may disturb rapid-eyeball-movement sleep.
5. does not produce dependence.

All benzodiazepines have anticonvulsant, muscle relaxant, anxiolytic and sedative–hypnotic activity and cause amnesia. The balance between these actions is said to vary in the different compounds. Thus **diazepam** is marketed primarily as an anxiolytic, **nitrazepam** and **flurazepam** as hypnotics and **clobazam** as an antiepileptic drug.

When the benzodiazepines are used as sedative–hypnotic drugs, tolerance, dependence and disturbances in rapid-eyeball-movement sleep are all seen, though to a smaller extent than with barbiturates. Long-term use in some elderly patients may result in drug cumulation and therefore a very prolonged sedative effect. Some patients find **nitrazepam** less effective than barbiturates in inducing sleep. The prime advantage of benzodiazepines is their relatively low toxicity and wide safety margin. It is difficult, though not impossible, to take a fatal overdose of **nitrazepam**. **Midazolam** is a newer, short-acting benzodiazepine, which is water-soluble and therefore can be given i.v. without causing pain or irritation.

Sleep comes on about 30 min after a hypnotic dose of **nitrazepam** and lasts 6–8 h. There is less hangover the following morning than with barbiturates and less impairment of fine skills. The interaction with **ethanol** is less marked but it is always best to instruct patients to avoid the combination of **alcohol** and hypnotic drugs. Indeed, **ethanol** itself (often in the form of whisky) may be an effective way of encouraging the onset of sleep in the elderly. Since many cases of insomnia are due to anxiety, the anxiolytic action of the benzodiazepines may help patients fall asleep.

Long-term therapy with benzodiazepines is viewed with suspicion since a variety of unwanted effects have been reported, especially in elderly patients. The incidence of these effects needs further investigation.

TTTTF

Some benzodiazepines and their uses

Drug and half-life	Uses	Comments
Flurazepam (S)	Hypnotic	Active metabolite (L)
Midazolam (S)	Sedative/preanaesthetic medication (i.v.)	Water-soluble
Temazepam (I)	Hypnotic	—
Nitrazepam (L)	Hypnotic	—
Clonazepam (L)	Antiepileptic	Slow tolerance
Diazepam (L)	Anxiolytic/status epilepticus/ preanaesthetic medication	Active metabolite (L)

Half-lives S = <6 h; I = 6–20 h; L = >20 h

MCQ 140

Regarding epilepsy,

1. grand mal, alone or in combination with other types of epilepsy, accounts for over 70% of cases.
2. grand mal attacks last less than 15 s.
3. petit mal occurs more commonly in children.
4. disturbances that are confined to the temporal region are termed psychomotor epilepsy.
5. attacks may be precipitated by flashing lights.

Epilepsy appears in a variety of forms and affects about 1 in 200 of the population. All types involve recurrent disturbances of brain activity, which may be symptomless (detected by EEG) or involve motor, sensory and/or psychic disturbances. Classically, in a grand mal attack, an initial transient 'aura' is followed by a tonic convulsion, in which all muscles contract and consciousness is lost. The patient falls to the ground and after 15–60 s exhibits a clonic convulsion, where major groups of muscles contract and relax alternately. Clonic movements of the jaw and lips cause the saliva to froth (frothing at the mouth) and there is urinary and faecal incontinence. After about 1–2 min the convulsion ceases, but the patient may remain unconscious for up to 1 h. On recovery there is usually confusion and total amnesia about the episode. Not all these stages are always present in every attack.

Petit mal is characterized by the brevity of the attacks. They may simply involve a clouding of consciousness for a few seconds and are then termed 'absences'. There are no convulsions but up to 100 absences may occur each day. Other types also exist, like focal epilepsy or psychomotor epilepsy, where the disturbance is confined to a particular area of the cortex or to the temporal region, respectively. Mixed types are common.

Attacks are associated with a spreading abnormal electrical discharge, initiated at a focus in the brain. The type and extent of symptoms depend on which particular areas are involved.

No consistent biochemical defect has been demonstrated. Birth injury, brain neoplasm, brain trauma and infection increase the likelihood of epilepsy. In a susceptible individual, attacks may be spontaneous but can be precipitated by flashing lights, exhaustion, overbreathing and stress. These factors are used in diagnosis when attacks are sometimes induced under controlled conditions. Diagnosis of the type of epilepsy is important as drugs may selectively benefit certain classes of epileptic patient only.

Uncontrolled epilepsy is debilitating and can severely interfere with patient and family. In children, petit mal can cause severe learning difficulties at school. Treatment does not cure the condition; it merely controls the symptoms. Cures do occur, but are more likely to be spontaneous than drug-induced. TFTTT

Of the antiepileptic drugs

1. **phenytoin** may produce gingival hyperplasia.
2. **phenytoin** may exacerbate petit mal.
3. **carbamazepine** has a tricyclic structure.
4. **sulthiame** interferes with the biotransformation of **phenytoin**.
5. most types can be detected by their effect on **strychnine**-induced convulsions in mice.

Phenytoin is frequently used as an antiepileptic agent, being particularly effective against grand mal and psychomotor epilepsy, but it will make petit mal worse. There is a non-linear relationship between the dose administered and the plasma levels of **phenytoin** which, together with the variation in sensitivity between patients, necessitates caution in its use. It is often useful therefore to measure *free* **phenytoin** in the plasma to ensure that satisfactory levels are being attained. Nausea, dizziness, skin rashes and vitamin D deficiency are all common side-effects. Overgrowth of the gums (gingival hyperplasia) until they cover the teeth and come into contact with the biting surfaces is one unusual side-effect seen with **phenytoin**.

Carbamazepine is a tricyclic drug similar in structure to the tricyclic antidepressants. However, it shows little antidepressant activity although dry mouth (frequently associated with antidepressants) is a common side-effect. It is useful in some resistant cases of grand mal or psychomotor epilepsy. **Carbamazepine** is also used in the treatment of trigeminal neuralgia, where the severe pain can be eased by the drug's ability to inhibit the generation and spread of electrical discharges in the trigeminal nerve.

Sulthiame has minimal antiepileptic action in its own right but potentiates the actions of **phenytoin** by reducing biotransformation. It is used, mainly in conjunction with **phenytoin**, against myoclonic and psychomotor epilepsy and side-effects include ataxia, anorexia, weight loss and psychic changes.

Initial screening of potential antiepileptic drugs is done almost exclusively in mice against electrical- or **leptazole**-induced convulsions. **Strychnine** causes convulsions by acting at a spinal level (it antagonizes the inhibitory spinal transmitter glycine) and is not a good model for epilepsy, which is a cortical disorder. In further tests, audiogenic seizures in rats can be used; or epilepsy may be induced by application of irritant material to the cortex. It is insufficient merely to establish pharmacological effectiveness; chronic toxicity must be very low as these agents may be given for years to epileptic patients. TTTTF

MCQ 142

Phenobarbitone, *when used as an antiepileptic agent, may*

1. induce rickets.
2. cause sedation.
3. cause skin reactions.
4. produce blood dyscrasias.
5. be contraindicated in patients suffering from defects in porphyrin metabolism.

Antiepileptic treatment is usually long term and sedation (to be expected with a barbiturate) occurs, especially at the start of treatment with **phenobarbitone**. Tolerance may later develop towards the sedation but to a lesser extent towards the antiepileptic effect, which suggests that different mechanisms are responsible for each effect. This hypothesis gains support from the fact that a different ratio exists between the antiepileptic and the sedative dose of many barbiturates. **Phenobarbitone** is particularly effective against grand mal and psychomotor epilepsy.

Liver microsomal enzymes are induced by **phenobarbitone** and therefore many drug interactions are caused by **phenobarbitone** altering the bio-transformation of other drugs. Cytochrome P-450 is also induced by **phenobarbitone**. The haem groups of the P-450 are generated by induction of the mitochondrial enzyme γ-aminolaevulinic acid synthetase. This is the rate-limiting step in the synthesis of the porphyrins used to produce haem. In normal patients the induction is of little importance but, in patients with a defect in porphyrin metabolism (e.g. acute intermittent porphyria), the accumulation of haem precursors in the blood can produce severe pain, gastrointestinal distress, nerve damage, psychic changes and even death. Defects in porphyrin metabolism may completely contraindicate barbiturates.

The enzymes responsible for the destruction of **vitamin D** are also induced and plasma **vitamin D** levels fall. Where **vitamin D** levels are already marginal, there may now be insufficient to allow complete calcification of bone (the resulting flexible skeletal structures will deform, giving the characteristic bow legs of rickety children). In adults the condition is known as osteomalacia and gives rise to spontaneous fractures and considerable pain.

Low serum **folate** levels are also produced by chronic **phenobarbitone** treatment. **Folate** is the precursor of tetrahydrofolate, which is crucial for the synthesis of purines and pyrimidines needed, for example, in the production of 10–20 g of red blood cells per day. In the absence of **folate**, megaloblasts are formed in the bone marrow and give rise to macrocytic rather than normal erythrocytes (hence megaloblastic macrocytic anaemia). Administration of **folate** supplements may prevent the foetal abnormalities and megaloblastic anaemia which could otherwise occur. However, the administration of large doses of **folate** may reduce the antiepileptic effectiveness of not only **phenobarbitone** but also **phenytoin**. TTTTT

The antiepileptic agent **sodium valproate**

1. produces respiratory depression.
2. is given orally to treat status epilepticus.
3. potentiates other antiepileptic agents.
4. produces nausea and sedation.
5. makes petit mal worse.

Sodium valproate is one of the most widely used antiepileptic agents, especially in new patients. It affects most types of epilepsy and has minimal side-effects. Sedation frequently occurs though this is usually mild and often disappears when treatment is maintained. Some patients complain of nausea but this is not severe.

Control of epilepsy may be achieved by any of several drugs, the choice being determined by the extent of undesirable effects produced at the required therapeutic dosage (i.e. therapeutic cost). On this basis **sodium valproate** appears to be superior to many other agents in that the incidence of undesirable effects is low and those which do occur are generally not very objectionable to the patient. Although other antiepileptic drugs are potentiated, **sodium valproate** is usually given alone in accordance with the present trend not to use combinations of antiepileptic drugs.

The great interest in **sodium valproate** lies in its close structural relationship to γ-aminobutyric acid (GABA), a known inhibitory transmitter in the CNS. This similarity fed speculation that antiepileptic drugs could act through an effect on GABA systems. **Sodium valproate** can inhibit GABA transaminase; the concentration of GABA in the brain may, therefore, be increased since this enzyme inactivates GABA.

Repeated grand mal attacks without recovery of consciousness between each episode constitute status epilepticus. It is a medical emergency and must be treated promptly and effectively otherwise death may result from anoxia, hyperpyrexia and exhaustion. Since the patient is unconscious, drugs cannot be swallowed and in any case would be absorbed too slowly. Administration i.v. produces an almost immediate effect though some drugs can be given i.m. when their action is nearly as fast. The treatment usually comprises i.v. administration of benzodiazepines like **diazepam** or **nitrazepam**, of **phenobarbitone** or of general anaesthetics. FFTTF

MCQ 144

Behavioural tests in rodents indicate that

1. a taming effect is produced by both major and minor tranquillizers.
2. **chlorpromazine** may inhibit conditioned avoidance responses without affecting escape responses.
3. barbiturates cannot be distinguished from major tranquillizers in such tests.
4. **haloperidol** causes catalepsy.
5. **amphetamine** induces stereotyped behaviour patterns.

Behavioural tests in rats are used extensively in the screening of psychoactive drugs. Spontaneous aggression (as exhibited by Rhesus monkeys or Siamese fighting fish) or induced aggression in rats or mice is decreased by both major and minor tranquillizers and these drugs are highly effective in producing a taming effect. Both groups of drugs also reduce spontaneous motor activity and potentiate the effects of other CNS depressants (e.g. barbiturates). However, all forms of behaviour are not affected equally by psychoactive drugs, and this is the basis of many screening tests.

For example, application through the cage floor of an electric shock will produce an 'escape response'; the rat tries to get away from the shock. If only part of the cage floor is electrified, the animal will quickly learn to escape to the 'safe' part of the cage when the shock is applied. If a conditioning stimulus (bell, light or buzzer) is given just before the shock, the rat will learn to associate the two stimuli and will move to the safe part of the cage on presentation of the conditioning stimulus thus avoiding completely the electric shock. The response to the conditioning stimulus is now a *'conditioned* avoidance' response. Major tranquillizers (e.g. **chlorpromazine**) inhibit the conditioned avoidance response in doses which do not block the escape response to the shock. Barbiturates, by contrast, will only disrupt the conditioned avoidance response in doses which inhibit the direct response to the shock and which produce frank ataxia.

Haloperidol, like many major tranquillizers, can induce catalepsy in high doses. Rats become immobile and will remain in any position (however bizarre) in which they are gently placed. The animals will still move if subjected to a painful stimulus, indicating that the muscular system and its direct control are still intact and that the rats still experience pain.

Amphetamine (a psychostimulant) greatly increases motor movements and causes stereotyped behaviour, for example compulsive gnawing or chewing in rats. **Amphetamine** injected into rats with a unilateral lesion on the nigrostriatal pathway causes the animal to turn, the circling movement being in the opposite direction from the lesioned side of the brain. This effect occurs because receptors in the CNS are stimulated by dopamine which **amphetamine** releases from intact neurones. By contrast, drugs stimulating the receptors directly (e.g. **bromocriptine**) will affect predominantly the supersensitive cell bodies which have been denervated and therefore cause rotation in the opposite direction (i.e. towards the lesion). TTFTT

Diazepam, chlordiazepoxide *and* phenobarbitone *all*

1. may be used as anxiolytic agents.
2. have sedative actions.
3. increase spontaneous motor activity.
4. have anticonvulsant activity.
5. selectively reduce polysynaptic reflex actively in the spinal cord.

All drugs with sedative actions can reduce feelings of anxiety, though the benzodiazepine tranquillizers **diazepam** and **chlordiazepoxide** have a separate, additional anxiolytic effect. This extra component is not present in barbiturates. The taming effect of benzodiazepines in aggressive animals is thought to be related to the more specific anxiolytic action in man. The sedative effect of benzodiazepines will reduce spontaneous motor activity but high doses are necessary. Both of these tranquillizers (and the related benzodiazepines **oxazepam**, **lorazepam** and **medazepam**) are centrally acting muscle relaxants (i.e. cause a selective reduction of polysynaptic reflex activity at the level of the spinal cord). They do not affect transmission or function in somatic cholinergic nerves.

All three drugs have anticonvulsant actions. **Phenobarbitone** is given for grand mal and other forms of epilepsy including status epilepticus (repeated grand mal seizures without recovery of consciousness in between). **Chlordiazepoxide** is rarely used in the chronic therapy of epilepsy, but **diazepam** is used mainly in status epilepticus and may well be the drug of choice in this condition. Other benzodiazepines like **clonazepam** or **clobazam** are more commonly used in the chronic treatment of epilepsy. However, as is the case with nearly all benzodiazepines, tolerance develops, though more slowly with this pair of drugs.

The above effects are shown by all benzodiazepines, though **nitrazepam**, **temazepam** and **flurazepam** tend to be used as hypnotic agents to produce sleep rather than to relieve anxiety during the day. While it is undoubtedly true that the benzodiazepines are relatively safe drugs in terms of acute overdose, it is clear that a considerable degree of dependence can be produced and that, especially in elderly patients, the drugs cumulate in the body during prolonged therapy.

Because of the dependence, patients experience great problems when they stop using benzodiazepines. Support groups which encourage self-help have been set up in many areas in attempts to benefit individuals trying to give up tranquillizers. TTFTF

MCQ 146

Both major and minor tranquillizers

1. produce sedation.
2. have antineurotic effects.
3. have antipsychotic effects.
4. are neuroleptics.
5. are effective in the treatment of schizophrenia.

Major and minor tranquillizers, exemplified by **chlorpromazine** and **diazepam** respectively, are used to treat mental illness. There are few clear-cut divisions between types of mental illness but it is helpful to distinguish two major groups, *neuroses* and *psychoses*. Generally, the neurotic patient shows a normal pattern of behaviour to an abnormal degree and is aware of his illness, i.e. has 'insight'. Anxiety, fear of confined spaces, sadness and self-criticism are normal feelings but, if carried to an extent that interferes with normal life, they become anxiety neurosis, claustrophobia and neurotic depression respectively. Between 2 and 10% of the population are thought to suffer from some form of neurosis and minor tranquillizers (**diazepam**, **chlordiazepoxide**) are usually given, though major tranquillizers are also effective.

The psychotic person shows behaviour patterns which are not seen in normal individuals (e.g. hallucinations), but lacks insight (awareness) that the behaviour is unusual. Examples of psychoses are schizophrenia and also affective disorders, like manic-depressive illness or severe depression accompanied by suicidal thoughts. Affective disorders are usually treated with antidepressants, but major tranquillizers and sometimes **lithium** salts are used in mania.

Schizophrenia is a complex disorder of thought, will, emotion and body movements. Delusions, fantasies and hallucinations are common. Emotions are blunted and the mood tends to be impassive. Body movements are abnormal and there may be overactivity, or lack of coordination or even catatonia (immobility and loss of responsiveness). There are spontaneous remissions from the acute symptoms and the incidence of schizophrenia within the population is about 1%.

The symptoms of a psychosis may be controlled by major tranquillizers (also called neuroleptics, psycholeptics or psychoplegics) but not by minor tranquillizers (psychosedatives, ataractics or anxiolytics). Sedation is frequently produced by both types of drug, reflecting their depressant effects on the CNS. However, for some patients the sedative effects may be useful (e.g. in conditions associated with agitation).

Mental disease is rarely *cured* by drugs – more usually therapy controls symptoms, though spontaneous remissions can occur, which may be prolonged. In addition, drugs may enable psychotherapy to be carried out more successfully. TTFFF

Schizophrenia

1. is treated with drugs which block central dopamine receptors.
2. may be treated using the phenothiazines **sulpiride** and **clozapine**.
3. usually responds immediately if neuroleptic drugs are given i.v.
4. involves thought disorders, hallucinations and delusions.
5. is usually accompanied by a movement disorder resembling parkinsonism.

Schizophrenia is a chronic psychiatric condition affecting about 1% of the population. It is manifested as disorders of thought, delusions, hallucinations and withdrawal from society. In general, patients are unaware of how different their behaviour is from the norm. The disease is progressive in nature and long-term drug treatment does not effect a cure. Theories on its cause are numerous; they have arisen after studying body fluids and tissues from patients or postmortem materials for biochemical and pathological changes; studies of the actions of drugs used to treat schizophrenia (neuroleptics) have also contributed to the theories. Most credence is given to the dopamine theory, which links the disorder to a change in the functional availability of this amine. Dopamine receptors have been subdivided into D_1 (functions uncertain but linked to adenyl cyclase), D_2 (principally found postsynaptically, not associated with adenylate cyclase, blocked by most neuroleptics) and D_3 (presynaptic, autoinhibitory).

Neuroleptic drugs fall into three major chemical groups:

(a) phenothiazines (e.g. **chlorpromazine**) and related compounds such as thioxanthenes (e.g. **flupenthixol**) or dibenzodiazepines (e.g. **clozapine**);
(b) butyrophenones (e.g. **haloperidol**);
(c) benzamides (e.g. **sulpiride**).

These drugs share the apparently crucial property of antagonizing dopamine, but their varying ability to affect other types of receptors may contribute to their undesirable effects (many phenothiazines block muscarinic cholinoceptors thereby causing, for example, dry mouth and blurred vision). The majority of neuroleptic drugs block both D_1- and D_2-dopamine receptors (the latter being more important clinically though, for example, **sulpiride** is more selective for D_2-receptors).

Side-effects of neuroleptic drugs are common and may be debilitating. Many are the consequence of D_2-receptor blockade in other parts of the CNS not associated with schizophrenia and are therefore predictable. For instance, D_2-receptors on prolactin-secreting pituitary cells are stimulated by endogenous dopamine, which inhibits prolactin output. This tonic suppression is lost when the receptors are blocked so that, during neuroleptic treatment, prolactin plasma levels rise leading, for example, to breast enlargement in men and inappropriate lactation in women. Furthermore, most neuroleptics cause an extrapyramidal syndrome (EPS) resembling Parkinson's disease by blocking D_2-receptors in the basal

continued on next page 179

ganglia. Least likely to provoke EPS are phenothiazines such as **thioridazine**, which has potent atropinic actions that help to counteract the EPS caused by D_2-receptor blockade, but in turn this leads to a higher incidence of unwanted effects like dry mouth and blurred vision. Surprisingly, the D_2-receptor blocker **sulpiride** is reported to be virtually devoid of EPS activity.

While the antagonism of dopamine occurs almost immediately, the clinical effects of neuroleptics are delayed by days or even weeks. The reasons are not fully understood but may be associated with an initial increase in activity of some central dopaminergic pathways which later wanes. In the longer term, an increase in the number of dopamine receptors occurs (such as is seen during 'denervation supersensitivity' phenomena). TFFTF

Chlorpromazine *used clinically may produce*

1. the same spectrum of effects as **promethazine**.
2. its full antipsychotic effect within a few hours of the first oral dose.
3. drowsiness and a fall in body temperature.
4. constipation and blurred vision.
5. postural hypotension and nasal stuffiness.

Chlorpromazine is the prototype major tranquillizer (neuroleptic), while **promethazine** is primarily antihistaminic. Both drugs are phenothiazines, **chlorpromazine** having a three-carbon chain between the phenothiazine nucleus and the attached amino group, **promethazine** having a two-carbon chain.

The full antipsychotic action of **chlorpromazine** is not brought about immediately after treatment begins. Improvement should be seen in 3 weeks, but it may take up to 6 weeks for the full therapeutic effect to develop. **Promethazine** does not have antipsychotic actions but both drugs produce sedation.

Blockade of dopamine receptors may be involved in the production of the antipsychotic effect of **chlorpromazine** and is certainly responsible for the antiemetic actions, the extrapyramidal signs (movement disorders) and the endocrine disturbances. Liberated from hypothalamic neurones, dopamine (now considered to be prolactin release inhibiting hormone) acts on D_2-receptors on pituitary cells to suppress prolactin output. If dopamine receptors are blocked, the levels of prolactin will increase, leading to gynaecomastia (breast growth) in men and galactorrhoea (lactation) in women. Pituitary gonadotrophin production is also disturbed and ovulation and menstruation are affected when dopamine receptors are blocked.

Chlorpromazine also blocks α-adrenoceptors, causing postural hypotension and nasal stuffiness. It blocks receptors for 5-hydroxytryptamine, leading to a fall in body temperature due to interference with the hypothalamic temperature-regulating centre. **Chlorpromazine** has atropinic actions causing reduced gastrointestinal motility, constipation, dry mouth, difficulty in initiating micturition and blurred vision. The drug also has a local anaesthetic effect and so may depress atrioventricular nodal conduction, leading to cardiac dysrhythmias. There is an adrenergic neurone blocking action and a blockade of noradrenaline reuptake. To what extent these actions contribute to the postural hypotension is unclear. Purple skin discolouration and rashes are also seen. Jaundice is common with long-term therapy.

It has been said that the trade name of the drug, 'Largactil', was derived from the large number of actions which **chlorpromazine** possesses. FFTTT

MCQ 149

The neuroleptic drug, haloperidol

1. is a phenothiazine like **droperidol** and **spiperone**.
2. is less potent in blocking α-adrenoceptors than is **chlorpromazine**.
3. causes less severe extrapyramidal effects than does **chlorpromazine**.
4. reduces serum prolactin levels.
5. has pronounced antidepressant properties.

Chemically, **haloperidol**, **spiperone** and **droperidol** are butyrophenones, not phenothiazines, though they share many of the pharmacological properties of the neuroleptic phenothiazines. For instance, **haloperidol** is a dopamine receptor blocking agent and has a potent antipsychotic effect. As with **chlorpromazine**, the dopamine receptor blockade will produce increased prolactin levels (leading to gynaecomastia and galactorrhoea), an antiemetic effect (through the chemoreceptor trigger zone) and the classical extra-pyramidal syndrome. The latter is particularly severe, since **haloperidol** has little compensatory atropinic activity which would return the disturbed dopamine–acetylcholine balance towards normal. However, this low atropinic activity results in only a limited disturbance of autonomic function. Interference with α-adrenoceptor function is also less marked than with **chlorpromazine**, so there is a lower incidence of hypotension and nasal stuffiness. **Haloperidol** does not have antidepressant properties but, like all antipsychotic agents, it is effective against the manic phase of manic-depressive illness. The closely related compound **droperidol** is used

(a) in anaesthetic practice in conjunction with the major narcotic analgesic **fentanyl** to induce 'neurolept analgesia';
(b) as an antiemetic premedication before surgical procedures;
(c) to prevent the hallucinations which frequently occur when adults emerge from **ketamine** anaesthesia.

Spiperone is also a butyrophenone and is an exceedingly potent antipsychotic drug. Its relatively high selectivity and affinity for dopamine receptors explains its common use as a ligand in binding studies to investigate and characterize dopamine receptors. FTFFF

The antiemetic action of chlorpromazine

1. occurs by depression of the chemoreceptor trigger zone in the medulla.
2. is utilized in the treatment of motion sickness.
3. is effective against **apomorphine**-induced vomiting.
4. is similar to that of **metoclopramide** and **promethazine**.
5. is effective against 'morning sickness' in pregnancy.

Apomorphine induces vomiting by stimulating dopamine receptors in the chemoreceptor trigger zone (CTZ) located in the area postrema of the medulla. At this site the blood–brain barrier is more permeable than normal and drug molecules penetrate the brain more readily. Not all phenothiazines are equally effective at blocking these dopamine receptors in the CTZ but **chlorpromazine, trifluoperazine, promazine** and **prochlorperazine** work well. They are all effective in reducing sickness due either to radiation or to drugs like **morphine**, oestrogens, tetracyclines and anticancer agents. Motion sickness is not affected to a great extent and, to treat this, other drugs are preferred which do not act on the CTZ (**promethazine, cyclizine** and **diphenhydramine** for example). Sickness in pregnancy is reduced by **chlorpromazine**, but it is best not to give *any* drugs during pregnancy unless they are essential. If drugs must be used, **chlorpromazine** is certainly not the drug of choice.

Some phenothiazines are occasionally used preoperatively as antiemetic agents and sedatives, although the newer halogenated hydrocarbon anaesthetics are less likely to produce vomiting than are the older agents. **Chlorpromazine** is rarely used since its hypotensive effect is very marked. Even with other phenothiazines there is a high incidence of unwanted effects and other types of drug are usually preferred.

Metoclopramide blocks dopamine receptors and shows many of the effects of **chlorpromazine** though it is less sedative. It is used to combat both motion sickness and the vomiting associated with some forms of cancer chemotherapy. In addition it stimulates gastric emptying without increasing HCl secretion, probably mediated indirectly by activating cholinergic nerves or possibly by blockade of 5-hydroxytryptamine (5-HT) receptors of the 5-HT$_3$ type. The effects appear to predominate in the upper part of the gastrointestinal tract, so **metoclopramide** is used to treat disorders of gastric emptying, or gastro-oesophageal reflux, or to aid ulcer healing. The research compound **GR38032F** is a potent antagonist at 5-HT$_3$ receptors and also increases gastric emptying. Because it lacks dopamine receptor blocking activity, it or related compounds could offer advantages over **metoclopramide** in the treatment of gastric disorders.

Promethazine is primarily an antihistamine drug and does not block dopamine receptors but commonly causes sedation. It is effective against motion sickness and in treating disturbances of the labyrinth (such as Ménière's syndrome). **Promethazine** can be used in 'morning sickness' but, as emphasized previously, it is better to avoid all drugs if possible during pregnancy. TFTFT

MCQ 151

The extrapyramidal symptoms induced by neuroleptic agents

1. may resemble Parkinson's disease.
2. are more often seen with **trifluoperazine** than with **pimozide**.
3. may be treated with **benzhexol** or **benztropine**.
4. result from a loss of dopamine from the substantia nigra.
5. are irreversible.

Four types of extrapyramidal syndrome may be caused by antipsychotic drugs. One develops slowly, after long-term therapy (tardive dyskinesia). The other types develop earlier during drug administration and are

(a) dystonia (facial grimaces and eye rolling);
(b) akathisia (restlessness and a compulsion to move around without purpose);
(c) a syndrome practically identical to Parkinson's disease.

Parkinson's disease is characterized by rigidity of skeletal muscles, movement disorders, tremor and infrequency of spontaneous movements. It is usually caused by degenerative changes in the dopaminergic neurones whose cell bodies lie in the substantia nigra. There is a consequential lack of dopaminergic control in the basal ganglia, where these neurones terminate. Since the effects of cholinergic and dopaminergic neurones are mutually antagonistic in the central control of fine movement, there is an apparent predominance of cholinergic activity when dopaminergic function is decreased.

Major tranquillizers, by blocking dopamine receptors (though leaving dopamine *levels* unchanged), produce a similar picture but not all major tranquillizers do so to a similar degree. Some of these drugs have prominent atropinic actions and, since it is the *balance* between cholinergic and dopaminergic function which is important, these drugs are less likely to cause the parkinsonian syndrome. Piperidyl phenothiazines (**thioridazine**, **mepazine**) are probably least likely to induce extrapyramidal signs. By contrast, piperazine phenothiazines (**fluphenazine, trifluoperazine**) do so frequently, some 40% of treated patients suffering these unwanted effects. The balance between cholinergic and dopaminergic activity also explains why these extrapyramidal effects can be treated with atropinic agents such as **benzhexol** or **benztropine**. **Sulpiride**, a benzamide, is a drug producing a low incidence of extrapyramidal effects, though the reasons are unclear.

Pimozide is an exceedingly potent dopamine receptor blocking agent with a low incidence of extrapyramidal side-effects. The reason for this is unclear since **pimozide** does not appear to exert atropinic actions. TTTFF

Tardive dyskinesia

1. is a neurological syndrome associated with prolonged use of minor tranquillizers.
2. involves repetitive movements of the tongue, jaw and lips.
3. is an iatrogenic disease.
4. may be persistent.
5. can be effectively treated by antiparkinsonian drugs.

Tardive dyskinesia is associated with prolonged antipsychotic drug use and is not seen with the minor tranquillizers. The syndrome involves involuntary sucking and smacking of the lips, sideways movements of the jaw and fast movements of the tongue. The syndrome is induced by drug therapy and is, therefore, an iatrogenic disease the incidence of which may be as high as 20% in some long-term psychiatric institutions. Once produced, the condition may be permanent. Treatment with antipsychotic drugs must be so organized as to reduce its occurence to a minimum.

The syndrome bears some resemblance to Parkinson's disease and lesions have been detected in the substantia nigra of patients with tardive dyskinesia. This area contains the dopaminergic pathways, degeneration of which leads to parkinsonism. Although its causes are not understood, tardive dyskinesia has been associated with the development of super-sensitivity to dopamine and with dysfunctions in γ-aminobutyric acid transmission in the substantia nigra. Unlike Parkinson's disease, however, tardive dyskinesia does not respond to treatment with **levodopa** and the use of atropinic drugs like **benzhexol** and **benztropine** is not always successful.

The syndrome is insidious (in that its appearance may be masked during administration of high doses of an antipsychotic drug) and only becomes apparent when the drug is withdrawn or the doses reduced. Prevention of the occurence of tardive dyskinesia is a major consideration in the design of antipsychotic therapy. The minimum adequate dose of drug should be used for the shortest period possible. If extrapyramidal effects occur, it may be appropriate to exchange the drug with one less likely to produce these effects (e.g. **thioridazine**) rather than to give atropinic agents in attempts to restore the dopamine–acetylcholine balance. FTTTF

MCQ 153

The movement disorder, parkinsonism

1. is caused by idiopathic degeneration of cholinergic neurones in the basal ganglia.
2. cannot be symptomatically improved by **dopamine** even when given intravenously.
3. has been treated by transplantation of brain tissue.
4. can be treated with phenothiazines like **ethopropazine**.
5. is cured by drugs like **bromocriptine** and **amantadine**.

Parkinsonism is an extrapyramidal tract disorder characterized by akinesia (reduced voluntary movements), rigidity and tremor. It is an idiopathic degenerative condition occurring especially in men of late middle age. A similar syndrome occurs in patients given certain phenothiazines and butyrophenones chronically, and also as an aftermath of the sleeping sickness (encephalitis lethargica) prevalent at the end of World War I. Postmortems on parkinsonian patients revealed degeneration of the dopaminergic nerves whose cell bodies were situated in the substantia nigra and terminals in the corpus striatum. Typically in such patients the innervated caudate nucleus contained very low levels of dopamine and it was reasoned that, if it could be replenished with the neurotransmitter, then symptomatic improvement, if not cure, would be brought about. **Dopamine** therapy was impractical since this amine will not penetrate to the striatum from the bloodstream. However, its immediate precursor, dopa, readily passes the blood–brain barrier on the amino acid carrier system. This substance (given orally as **levodopa**) proved an effective therapy for many parkinsonian patients, especially those who were not severely incapacitated by the disease.

Not all types of treatment were rationally developed. **Belladonna** extracts, used first in the late 19th century and, later, synthetic atropinic drugs were moderately successful, especially in reducing the tremors of Parkinson's disease. Indeed, atropinic drugs, such as **benztropine**, **trihexylphenidate** or **ethopropazine** (a phenothiazine), are often used, alone or in combination with other drugs, in the initial therapy of the disease. It is now understood that blockers of acetylcholine at central muscarinic receptors will reduce the unopposed cholinergic tone that results from depletion of the functionally antagonistic dopamine.

Other antiparkinsonian agents exist which have different mechanisms of action. **Bromocriptine**, which is an ergot derivative, has a direct stimulant effect on dopamine receptors. It is especially useful in patients coming off **levodopa** therapy and may be used in combination with the latter or other drugs. **Bromocriptine** is also used to treat endocrinological disorders like hyperprolactinaemia. **Amantadine** is an antiviral agent found by chance to be useful against parkinsonism. Its mode of action is uncertain though it probably influences the synthesis, release or neuronal reuptake of dopamine. The benefits are often short-lived, patients becoming refractory after a few months' treatment.

Interest has been aroused by a striking improvement in the condition of some parkinsonian patients who received implants of brain tissue removed from aborted foetuses. Ethical considerations have delayed wide trials of such therapy but more reports of the possible benefits and hazards are likely in the future. FTTTF

In the management of Parkinson's disease, **levodopa**

1. is often given with **carbidopa** to increase its effectiveness.
2. causes dyskinesias in a high proportion of patients, especially when administered with peripheral dopa decarboxylase inhibitors.
3. may be given simultaneously with **benserazide**, **amantadine** or with atropinic drugs.
4. may be administered along with a catechol-*O*-methyltransferase inhibitor, like **selegiline**, to reduce its toxicity.
5. may cause depression, cardiac dysrhythmias and hypertension.

The recognition that a central dopamine deficiency might be remedied by treatment with a precursor culminated in the introduction of **levodopa** for the treatment of parkinsonism in the 1960s. The amino acid is taken up by those remaining functional dopaminergic fibres of the degenerating nigrostriatal pathway. It also enters peripheral and central noradrenergic fibres, as well as those nerves which normally synthesize 5-hydroxytryptamine. In these latter neurones, dopamine will first be formed because they all possess the enzyme aromatic L-amino acid decarboxylase (commonly known as dopa decarboxylase). Many undesirable effects are associated with the biotransformation of large doses of **levodopa** in non-dopaminergic systems.

In attempts to reduce the incidence of unwanted effects (nausea and vomiting, cardiac dysrhythmias, hypertension and psychiatric disorders), lower doses (1 g or less) are now used. This has been made possible by the development of dopa decarboxylase inhibitors (**carbidopa**, **benserazide**) which themselves fail to penetrate the CNS. Given orally they block the conversion of **levodopa** to dopamine in the gut and liver, and also in peripheral catecholaminergic neurones. Thus, from a given dose of **levodopa**, a larger fraction will be available for uptake into the brain. Hence improvements of parkinsonism might be expected with fewer undesirable peripheral effects.

The monamine oxidase (MAO) inhibitor **selegiline** is presently being used in combination with reduced doses of **levodopa** to treat parkinsonism. Monoamine oxidase exists in two forms, types A and B, which have different substrate specificities, for example **tyramine** is biotransformed principally by MAO-A. Since **selegiline** is a selective inhibitor of MAO-B and acts to preserve CNS dopamine (formed from the **levodopa**), it can be safely used even if patients consume food containing large amounts of **tyramine**. A possible future development in therapy concerns inhibitors of catechol-*O*-methyltransferase (COMT), an enzyme which biotransforms **levodopa** especially when other pathways (e.g. dopa decarboxylase) are blocked. Presently restricted to animal studies, some new inhibitors of COMT have been shown to increase the levels of **levodopa** (given with **carbidopa**) both in the periphery and brain. It remains to be seen if clinical advances may result.

Nonetheless, the course of idiopathic parkinsonism is unaffected by drugs and the benefits with **levodopa** gradually diminish. Multiple therapy is common in the severest cases so that **levodopa**, **carbidopa**, **amantadine** and an atropinic drug may be given together. A majority of patients on long-term therapy (especially when **levodopa** is combined with **carbidopa**) suffer from dystonias, tics and dyskinesias like chorea. Sometimes periods without drugs may be helpful by reducing the behavioural side-effects and dyskinesias. TTTFT

Huntington's chorea involves a

1. single recessive gene and inheritance occurs in individuals who are homozygous.
2. loss of cells from the cortex, resulting in dementia.
3. loss of cells from the cerebellum, resulting in involuntary writhing movements.
4. reduction in dopamine in the striatum.
5. defect in copper metabolism.

Huntington's chorea is an inherited disease which usually becomes apparent between the ages of 20 and 50. It is inherited through a single autosomal dominant gene probably associated with a unique DNA sequence found on chromosome 4. This finding should allow the development of methods which will accurately predict the likelihood of an individual developing the disease. There will then be a good chance that the incidence of the disease can be reduced through genetic counselling, one of the most important aspects of the management of this distressing and progressive condition for which treatment is presently unsatisfactory. Behavioural changes eventually predominate but loss of cortical cells produces dementia and loss of cells from the striatum produces the chorea (involuntary irregular unpredictable movements which occur in one part of the body or another in unpredictable sequence).

Postmortem examination of brains has demonstrated that dopamine in the striatum is normal (thus differentiating this condition from Parkinson's disease) and that there is a large drop in striatal glutamic acid decarboxylase, the enzyme which synthesizes γ-aminobutyric acid (GABA). It is thought that the loss of GABA-mediated inhibition in the striatum leads to an overactivity of dopaminergic systems. Since there is also a loss of choline acetylase and underactivity of striatal cholinergic systems, Huntington's chorea is in a sense the opposite of Parkinson's disease, which involves underactivity of dopaminergic systems and relative overactivity of cholinergic systems. As might be expected, therefore, drugs beneficial in Parkinson's disease (**levodopa, bromocriptine**) exacerbate the chorea but dopamine antagonists (**haloperidol**) may produce some improvement. Attempts have been made to compensate for the GABA deficiency by using GABA transaminase inhibitors (**sodium valproate**) to prevent GABA breakdown but drugs generally do not affect the progressive nature of the disease, which is invariably fatal.

Wilson's disease is a consequence of a rare inherited recessive defect in copper metabolism which allows copper to accumulate in basal ganglia, cortex, liver and elsewhere. Typically, onset is early in life (before 15 years) and is characterized by a developing chorea, dementia and behavioural changes. The disease is treatable with oral **penicillamine** starting with a small dose and monitoring plasma copper levels. A low copper diet and zinc supplements may also help and once treatment has begun it will need to be continued for life. FTFFF

Tricyclic antidepressants

1. provide rapid relief from the symptoms of affective disorders.
2. reduce the pressor response to **tyramine**.
3. may promote the neuronal reuptake of 5-hydroxytryptamine and noradrenaline.
4. are exemplified by **mianserin**.
5. include dibenzazepines such as **imipramine**.

Affective disorders are *primarily* disturbances in mood (affect). Both endogenous and exogenous (reactive) types of depression fall into this category. Their symptoms are apathy, mental and physical slowing, sadness, self-deprecation, indifference, lack of energy, early morning wakening, loss of appetite and suicidal tendencies. Manic-depressive illness is also an affective disorder, involving swings of mood between mania (elation, hyperactivity, uncontrolled thought and speech) and depression. On the other hand, schizophrenia, paranoia and some movement disorders (e.g. Parkinson's disease) are not affective disorders since the changes in mood which occur are not the primary disorder.

Therapy of affective disorders may be pharmacological, using drugs such as monoamine oxidase inhibitors, tricyclic or the newer antidepressant drugs, or, in the case of manic-depressive psychosis, **lithium** salts may be given. Alternatively, electroconvulsive therapy may be employed. Psychotherapy is sometimes used in conjunction with these treatments and other psychoactive drugs may have a role.

The tricyclic antidepressants, as their name implies, have a common structural feature of three fused rings. Classical examples are **imipramine** and **amitriptyline** and their desmethyl analogues **desmethylimipramine** and **nortriptyline**. It should be noted that **imipramine** is a *di*benzazepine (meaning two phenyl (benzene) rings plus a seven-membered ring containing one nitrogen atom). It should not be confused with benzo*di*azepines, like **diazepam**, which possess a seven-membered ring containing *two* nitrogen atoms. Some of the newer antidepressants (e.g. **mianserin**) have a four-ring system and are not *tri*cyclic though they may have some similar properties.

All antidepressants affect monoamines in the CNS, especially 5-hydroxytryptamine (5-HT) and noradrenaline (NA). Generally, tricyclic antidepressants block the reuptake of NA and/or 5-HT into neurones, thereby increasing the availability of these amines within the synaptic cleft. Uptake blockade takes place within a few hours of the first dose but it may take as long as a month for the full therapeutic effect to develop. The reason for this delay is uncertain but may be related to a long-term regulation of the number of amine receptors. Because these drugs inhibit the reuptake of NA (uptake-1), they reduce the effects of indirectly acting sympathomimetic amines, like **tyramine**, which must be taken up into the neurone by uptake$_1$ before displacing NA. FTFFT

MCQ 157

Side-effects commonly associated with the use of tricyclic antidepressant drugs include

1. dry mouth.
2. sedation.
3. constipation and difficulty in initiating micturition.
4. blurred vision.
5. postural hypotension.

Atropine-like actions (antagonism of muscarinic actions of acetylcholine) are shown by many tricyclic antidepressant drugs. The salivary glands, bladder and intestinal muscles and ciliary muscles controlling visual accommodation are all cholinergically innervated and contain muscarinic receptors, so their functions are impaired. Some of the newer antidepressants like **mianserin** and **iprindole** are relatively free of atropinic effects and are generally preferred by patients, although blood dyscrasias have been reported in some patients given **mianserin**.

The commonly occurring sedation (seen in normal volunteers as well as in depressed patients) may become less marked as treatment progresses and can be made less objectionable if the main dose of the antidepressant is given at night rather than in the morning. By contrast, the monoamine oxidase inhibitors (alternative antidepressants) tend to have a stimulant or mood-elevating effect in normal individuals.

Postural hypotension (dizziness on rising due to decreased blood supply to the brain) may occur, due to α_1-adrenoceptor blockade at the arterioles. This reduces sympathetic vasoconstriction and thus inhibits cardiovascular compensatory reflexes. Alternatively, postural hypotension might result from an effect on cardiovascular controlling centres in the CNS.

The antidepressant effect of tricyclics is not seen until they have been given for 1–3 weeks but the above side-effects occur within 24 h of the first dose. This separation between onset of undesirable and beneficial effects may account for the very poor patient compliance. Patients simply stop taking the pills as they seem to be doing no good. It is wise to measure plasma antidepressant levels since a lack of response may simply be due to poor compliance.

Measurement of plasma levels is also useful because there are considerable differences in bioavailability of antidepressants between patients. Furthermore, there may be a 'therapeutic window', below or above which beneficial effects are not seen. Measurement of plasma levels permits the drug dosage to be adjusted to individual needs. TTTTT

Poisoning with tricyclic antidepressants is likely to

1. be rare.
2. be easily remedied.
3. involve coma and convulsions.
4. involve cardiac dysrhythmias.
5. involve raised blood pressure.

Individuals suffering from depressive illnesses may have suicidal tendencies and may make hysterical or serious suicide attempts. One readily available means of attempting suicide is by an overdose of drugs and antidepressants are frequently misused in this way. Mothers suffering from depression may uncaringly leave their tablets accessible to children, so this group is also at risk from poisoning. Of all deaths due to poisoning in the UK in 1982 more than 13% involved an antidepressant and in 1986 the figure had risen to about 18%, though it should not be inferred that the antidepressant was the cause of death in every case. This percentage is out of all proportion to the number of doses prescribed.

Treatment of poisoning is often difficult because in many suicide attempts several types of poison are taken at one time. In addition, the combination of toxic effects (convulsions, cardiac dysrhythmias, coma and cardiovascular problems) is difficult to control and no specific antidote is available.

A great variety of cardiac dysrhythmias may occur even up to several days after the toxic dose has been consumed. The cardiac effects may in part be due to blockade of noradrenaline uptake, thereby increasing the effectiveness of sympathetic stimulation to the heart. There may be another component, since many antidepressants directly affect cardiac conduction and excitability. The treatment is to limit further absorption of drug if possible (stomach wash), to monitor cardiac function and to treat symptomatically. The anticholinesterase **physostigmine** has some beneficial effects, although it is unclear whether they result from antagonism of the atropinic effects of the tricyclic antidepressants centrally and peripherally, or are caused by the accumulated acetylcholine acting as a functional antagonist. FFTTT

MCQ 159

Antidepressants of the monoamine oxidase inhibitor type

1. are more effective in endogenous than exogenous (reactive) depression.
2. produce a feeling of well-being in both depressed and normal individuals.
3. are likely to reduce blood pressure.
4. may cause dry mouth and constipation.
5. have a long duration of action but are rapid in onset.

Exogenous depression (also called 'reactive' because it has an identifiable outside cause, such as family bereavement) is reputed to respond more readily to monoamine oxidase inhibitors (MAOIs) than does endogenous depression, where no outside cause can be identified. By contrast with tricyclic antidepressants (which are sedative and do not elevate mood in normal individuals), the MAOIs elevate mood in both normal and depressed individuals. Some drugs inhibit monoamine oxidase competitively (**pargyline**) while others are non-competitive (**isocarboxazid, nialamide**). All have a long duration of action, taking about 1 week to be removed from the body.

Generally, they are non-specific in their action, inhibiting not only mitochondrial monoamine oxidase but also liver microsomal enzymes. Thus MAOIs potentiate the effects of a great variety of drugs by altering drug biotransformation. Blockade of monoamine oxidase in liver and in the gut wall is responsible for the potentiation of indirectly acting sympathomimetics, taken by mouth, like **tyramine**, that are normally rapidly deaminated by monoamine oxidase. The 'cheese reaction' in patients given MAOIs is a dangerous hypertensive state caused by potentiation of **tyramine** found in certain types of cheese. Cheese should be avoided (as should yeast extract and certain wines) when MAOIs are taken.

As with tricyclic antidepressants there is a delay of up to 28 days before the full therapeutic effect of MAOIs is seen. Dry mouth and constipation are frequent side-effects, probably due to a decreased cholinergic output from the CNS rather than peripheral atropinic activity. Hypotension is common and it should be noted that some of the MAOIs (**pargyline**) have been used as antihypertensive agents. The mechanisms involved are unclear but may involve a reduction in sympathetic ganglionic transmission.

Generally, the simultaneous use of tricyclic antidepressants and MAOIs is unwise as adverse reactions have been reported. However, on some occasions the combination has been used successfully.

Monoamine oxidase is not a homogenous enzyme and two types (A and B) are recognized, for which substrate specificities differ and for which selective inhibitors are known (e.g. **clorgyline** blocks MAO-A and **selegiline** MAO-B). Interestingly, **selegiline** is used as an adjunctive treatment in parkinsonism and acts by preserving central dopamine formed by concurrently administered **levodopa**. Since **tyramine** is a substrate for MAO-A, foods containing the amine can be safely eaten by patients taking **selegiline**. FTTTF

The antidepressant

1. **clorgyline** is a tricyclic antidepressant.
2. **imipramine** has very similar actions to **mianserin**.
3. **maprotiline** is a monoamine oxidase inhibitor.
4. effect of electroconvulsive therapy is seen after one application of electrical discharge to the temporal region of the head for 15 s.
5. **nialamide** is likely to produce hepatotoxic effects.

Clorgyline is a monoamine oxidase inhibitor (MAOI), not a tricyclic antidepressant drug. Monoamine oxidase exists as two isoenzymes (A and B) for which selective inhibitors are known; **clorgyline**, effective in the treatment of depression, is an MAO-A inhibitor. **Mianserin**, having a four-ring structure, is one of the newer antidepressant drugs. It has fewer atropinic effects than the older tricyclics and is less likely to disturb cardiac function. Since, in older patients, depression and abnormal cardiac function may coexist, this is an important advantage. Nonetheless, **mianserin** is not devoid of unwanted effects (e.g. blood dyscrasias have been reported). **Maprotiline** has a bismethylene bridge across the central ring and therefore is not strictly a tricyclic though it shares many of the properties of the tricyclic antidepressants. **Maprotiline** is not a MAOI.

Electroconvulsive therapy (ECT) involves the application, at intervals of a few days, of electrical shocks (of 0.1–0.6 s duration) to the temples. Several sessions may be needed before significant improvement is produced. Often ECT is given under light anaesthesia (**thiopentone**) and neuromuscular blockade (**succinylcholine**). Considerable controversy surrounds the use of ECT but nonetheless it may act more rapidly than drugs and may be effective in patients in whom drugs have failed.

Not all patients respond to ECT or to the tricyclic antidepressants. Subgroups of depressed patients may exist who respond better to one group of drugs than another. Thus there may be more than one biochemical defect underlying depression and this would explain why no completely satisfactory unifying theory of depression exists.

Most MAOIs, including **nialamide**, **isocarboxazid** and **phenelzine**, are not selective for types A and B. These belong to the hydrazine (−NH−NH−) group of drugs and none of them is *likely* to produce liver damage. The incidence of this problem is low (about 1%) but when it does occur the associated mortality is around 15%. Non-hydrazine MAOIs, like **pargyline** and **clorgyline**, have not been reported to cause hepatotoxicity. FFFFF

MCQ 161

Lithium, *used in the treatment of manic-depressive illness,*

1. is usually administered as the carbonate.
2. is effective within 3 days of beginning treatment.
3. is effective against the manic phase.
4. is effective against the depressive phase.
5. produces gastrointestinal and CNS side-effects.

Lithium bromide (note bromide toxicity) and **chloride** were used earlier to treat manic-depressive illness but **lithium carbonate** or **citrate** are always used nowadays. As with tricyclic antidepressants and monoamine oxidase inhibitors the therapeutic effect takes 1–4 weeks to develop fully, although this does not necessarily mean that the same mechanism of action is involved. Both phases of manic-depressive illness are reduced but **lithium** salts are less effective than other antidepressant drugs in the treatment of pure depression.

The mode of action of **lithium** is unclear. As a monovalent ion it can enter cells through Na^+ channels, especially in excitable cells where they are voltage-operated, but it is eliminated more slowly than sodium and therefore accumulates. An effect of **lithium** has been reported on the phosphatidyl inositol pathway which results in depletion of phosphatidyl inositol biphosphate in the membrane and an increase of cytosolic inositol-1-phosphate. In some cells **lithium** reduces the production of cyclic AMP brought about by hormone stimulation. The relevance of these findings to the use of **lithium** in psychiatry is unclear.

Two major groups of toxic effects are seen with **lithium carbonate**: first, gastrointestinal (pain, thirst, nausea, vomiting and diarrhoea) and, second, neurological (dizziness, tremor, slurred speech and muscle twitching). The therapeutic index of **lithium** is low and, while plasma levels of 0.5–1.5 mM are therapeutically effective, toxic symptoms appear at 2 mM and severe toxicity is exhibited at 3 mM. The dose regime is important and patients usually start with 2 g per day in divided doses until a response is seen. Then the dose is reduced to a maintenance level of 0.5–1 g per day. Routine measurement of **lithium** plasma levels is very useful.

Lithium is effective against acute mania whether given therapeutically or prophylactically. Treatment should be continued even after the acute manic state has passed. TFTTT

Morphine

1. like **papaverine**, is an analgesic alkaloid found in opium.
2. suppresses both the perception of and the reaction to pain without causing loss of consciousness.
3. has antitussive and antiemetic activity.
4. causes biliary duct spasm.
5. produces mydriasis by reducing activity in the parasympathetic nerves to the sphincter pupillae.

The juice which exudes from unripe seed capsules of the poppy *Papaver somniferum* hardens on exposure to air and is then called opium. This brown gum contains alkaloids of two chemical classes: the phenanthrene alkaloids like **morphine** and **codeine**, which are analgesic, and the benzoisoquinoline alkaloids like **papaverine** and **thebaine**, which are not.

Opium contains about 10% **morphine**, which is the most potent natural analgesic alkaloid. **Morphine** also possesses many other properties, some of which severely limit its application as a pain-killing drug (for example, both tolerance and dependence develop when the drug is used repeatedly). **Morphine** is often described as a 'narcotic analgesic' though the drug produces sedation in normal doses rather than the loss of consciousness implied by the term narcosis. The term is best avoided and we will use 'opioid' to distinguish morphine-like analgesics from the aspirin-like group.

Morphine interacts with receptors located in several areas of the brain and in the periphery to produce its actions, which include the following:

(a) suppression of both *perception* of and *reaction* to pain;
(b) euphoria, a freeing from anxiety and stress which occurs especially in patients who were in severe pain;
(c) sedation sufficient to bring about sleep, especially in the elderly, but without any amnesia;
(d) depression of the cough reflex (antitussive action) occasionally employed in patients with intractable cough;
(e) respiratory depression manifested by decreased responsiveness to carbon dioxide;
(f) nausea and vomiting mainly through an action on the chemoreceptor trigger zone, but vestibular effects may also contribute since the action is more marked in ambulant patients;
(g) constipation, most regions of the gastrointestinal tract showing reduced propulsive movements and, occasionally, increased resting muscle tone.
(h) abdominal pain from constriction of the bile duct and the sphincter of Oddi, thus raising biliary pressure;
(i) increased bladder and urethral muscle tone accompanied by constriction of sphincters, which may lead to retention of urine (e.g. postoperatively);
(j) pupillary constriction (miosis) causing 'pin-point pupils';
(k) inhibition of neuronally induced contraction of the vas deferens or small intestine in some species.

FTFTF

MCQ 163

Opioid peptides are

1. components of opioid receptors to which **morphine** binds.
2. molecules such as the pentapeptides methionine-enkephalin and leucine-enkephalin.
3. found both in the CNS and in the periphery.
4. found in precursor proteins which contain the corticotrophin (adrenocorticotrophic hormone) amino acid sequence.
5. antagonists of **morphine**.

The basis of **morphine**'s pharmacological action was discovered in the 1970s principally through the work of Hughes, Kosterlitz and their co-workers in the UK and of Snyder, Pert *et al.* in the USA. Receptors of several types are found both centrally and peripherally and are classified according to their interactions with exogenous and endogenous ligands. They have been studied by a variety of techniques (e.g. in the CNS by immunohistochemistry, radioligand binding and autoradiography). The distribution of these receptors is matched by the high concentrations of endogenous ligands found in the same locations. Various collective names have been proposed for the endogenous ligands, the least controversial being 'opioid peptides'.

The smallest peptides which bind to opioid receptors each possess five amino acids (methionine-enkephalin and leucine-enkephalin) and are found in the CNS in high concentration in the locality of opioid receptors. Despite being rapidly biotransformed *in vivo*, they produce analgesia when administered suitably and, given microiontophoretically to single neurones, they are generally depressant in areas thought to be associated with pain. Conflicting views have been expressed as to whether these pentapeptides are neurotransmitters with normal functions concerned with the suppression of pain.

Many other peptides bind to opioid receptors and possess opioid activity. Some may be precursors of the pentapeptide enkephalins and others may have neurotransmitter or neuromodulator roles in their own right. Certain large polypeptides (containing more than 250 amino acid units) yield fragments having the same amino acid sequences as are found in the enkephalins. A fragment containing 17 amino acids (dynorphin) is one of the most potent agonists at opioid receptors. An important precursor protein is pro-opiomelanocortin, which contains amino acid sequences not only of a major opioid (β-endorphin) but also of melanocyte-stimulating hormone and of corticotrophin (adrenocorticotrophic hormone). The presence and the properties of these related peptides suggest that a neurological system exists which selectively produces and uses opioid peptides.

Of the several types of opioid receptor the most important with regard to the actions of **morphine** are the mu receptors, which mediate respiratory depression, euphoria, supraspinal analgesia and physical dependence, and the kappa receptors, which mediate sedation, miosis and spinal analgesia.
FTTTF

Drugs which can be used clinically instead of morphine

1. include **methadone**, used to produce analgesia.
2. are all less potent but have fewer undesirable effects.
3. include **pethidine**, which is contraindicated in obstetrics since it crosses the placenta.
4. include substances which are partial agonists at opioid receptors, like **pentazocine**
5. include **naloxone**, which is a powerful analgesic with minimum liability to cause dependence.

Morphine is used for the suppression of severe pain and is better against constant rather than intermittent sharp pain. Pain associated with cancer and other terminal illnesses is relieved. Tolerance and dependence do not really present problems in terminal cases, where it is important to give enough drug, sufficiently often, to provide effective relief. A special use of i.v. **morphine** is in the relief of pulmonary oedema associated with left ventricular failure but the mechanisms involved are not clear.

Many attempts have been made to synthesize analgesics which lack the undesirable features of **morphine** (e.g. tolerance, dependence, respiratory depression). Complete separation of the beneficial and the unwanted effects of **morphine** has not been achieved but some compounds may possess clinical advantages in certain respects. **Methadone** has a longer duration of effect than **morphine** and is effective by mouth. Dependence and tolerance develop more slowly and the withdrawal syndrome is less intense. It is often substituted for **morphine** or **heroin** in attempts to wean addicts from these drugs.

Fentanyl is a potent morphine-like analgesic often used in operative procedures. Its strong respiratory depressant effect is less important under these conditions because respiration is usually supported since neuromuscular blocking agents will have been given. It is occasionally used in combination with the major tranquillizer **droperidol** to produce 'narcolept analgesia', where the pain of a surgical procedure is removed while the patient remains able to respond to commands.

Pethidine is widely used in obstetrics, especially during labour, since it crosses the placental barrier less well than **morphine** and produces less foetal respiratory depression.

Codeine is much less powerful than **morphine** with regard to the intensity of pain which can be relieved. It is often formulated as a mild analgesic with **aspirin** and/or **paracetamol** and in these combinations dependence is no problem. **Codeine** is a useful antitussive and will suppress the cough reflex at doses which produce little analgesia. **Dextromethorphan** and **pholcodine** are related, effective antitussive agents.

Pentazocine and some other benzomorphans have a mixed agonist–antagonist action and are less likely than **morphine** to produce dependence. **Meptazinol** is also less likely to produce dependence and is said to produce less respiratory depression at equivalent analgesic doses.

Acute opioid overdose can be treated with antagonists like **naloxone** or the longer-lasting **naltrexone**. TFFTF

MCQ 165

The withdrawal syndrome which occurs in an addict abstaining from heroin

1. begins with signs of sleeplessness, yawning and euphoria.
2. appears as overactivity of the sympathetic nervous system in the early stages.
3. may be minimized by first stabilizing the addict on orally administered **methadone**.
4. may last for 6 months.
5. may be minimized by treatment with **clonidine**.

Tolerance and dependence are associated with many drugs which have actions on the CNS. Dependence may be either 'psychic' or 'physical'. Psychic dependence is the compulsive drug-seeking behaviour seen in people who use drugs for personal satisfaction (e.g. the craving for **alcohol** or **nicotine**). Physical dependence involves the appearance of a characteristic withdrawal syndrome associated with changes in physiological functions which is seen when the drug is no longer available to the body. Barbiturates, opioids and benzodiazepines may all produce physical dependence to a greater or lesser extent.

Tolerance implies a decreased responsiveness to a drug, which can usually be counteracted by increasing the dose administered. It may be metabolic in origin, for example when a drug is more rapidly biotransformed by induced microsomal enzymes. Tolerance may be behavioural, where the individual learns, by modifying behaviour patterns, to operate normally even in the continued presence of the drug. Alternatively, tolerance may be induced by an alteration in the number of available receptors for the drug.

Dependence often results from the abuse of drugs such as the opioids, **cocaine** and barbiturates. In opioid abuse the drugs are nearly always given i.v. and produce euphoria, tranquillity and sleepiness. In the case of **heroin**, three or four daily doses are often needed to maintain the desired state, so that money (hence the link with crime) or supplies run out and the withdrawal syndrome starts. Typically this varies with the category of drug involved, but for the opioids the first signs are often increased sympathetic activity, running eyes and nose, sweating and yawning. Chills are experienced and goose-flesh is prominent, together with nausea and vomiting, cramp-like pains and extreme restlessness. This syndrome is characteristic of the acute phase of withdrawal, which is usually over within 3 weeks, but there is a secondary phase (involving hypotension, hypothermia and mydriasis) which may last 6 months.

Withdrawal is very unpleasant, especially if high doses of **heroin** have been used for long periods. Progressive substitution of **heroin** by **methadone** followed by withdrawal of **methadone** is much easier. Recently **clonidine** has been used to suppress withdrawal symptoms, presumably working because it suppresses the sympathetic overactivity associated with withdrawal since **clonidine** itself has no action on opioid receptors.

Once withdrawal is complete, psychotherapy, group therapy, meditation and changing the social environment may all play a role in discouraging a return to drug abuse. Nevertheless, the rate of complete cure is very low and up to 85% may become addicted again within 2 years. FTTTT

Drugs affecting the gastrointestinal tract include

1. **morphine**, which causes constipation.
2. **diphenoxylate**, a remedy for diarrhoea.
3. **pholcodine**, a purgative and antiemetic drug.
4. **bisacodyl**, an analogue of **codeine**, which relieves diarrhoea.
5. **cellulose**, a bulk-forming laxative.

Morphine and several structurally related drugs (e.g. **diphenoxylate**) have a constipating effect by reducing peristaltic activity. Although **diphenoxylate** is qualitatively similar to **morphine**, it is relatively more potent in its actions on the gut. However, it has a much lower incidence of producing dependence, partly because its insolubility makes it difficult for narcotic addicts to extract **diphenoxylate** from tablets. It is widely used as a remedy for diarrhoea, especially in combination with **atropine** (**Lomotil**).

Pholcodine is used primarily as an antitussive in doses which are unlikely to cause dependence but which do cause constipation.

While morphine-like drugs generally reduce gut activity, there is a wide variety of other agents which increase gut action. Laxatives ease the passage of stools and help patients who may otherwise produce rectal damage by straining at impacted stools. Laxatives may be bulk-forming (e.g. **cellulose**) or lubricating (e.g. **liquid paraffin**, which may be absorbed and accumulate in lymph glands and which may reduce the absorption of fat-soluble vitamins).

Purgatives cause evacuation of the bowel and can be used to remove poisons or to eliminate worms after anthelminthic therapy. Gut irritants have purgative effects (e.g. **castor oil**, which liberates the irritant ricinoleic acid; **senna**, **aloes** and **cascara**). Some irritate the colon, like **bisacodyl** and the related drug **phenolphthalein**. The action of the latter is prolonged because it enters the enterohepatic circulation.

In Western society there is excessive concern about bowel function. A sensible diet, including plenty of roughage, will eliminate the need for laxatives or purgatives other than in particular medical conditions. Whilst drugs may temporarily relieve the discomfort, inconvenience and danger associated with severe diarrhoea, their long-term use is ill-advised. The cause of the disorder should be discovered and treated rather than the symptoms.
TTFFT

Endocrine Pharmacology

The pituitary gland

1. is also called the hypophysis.
2. releases the peptide oxytocin from the posterior lobe.
3. secretes corticotrophin (adrenocorticotrophic hormone) when adeno-hypophyseal dopaminergic nerves are stimulated.
4. produces somatostatin, a physiological antagonist of growth hormone.
5. is innervated by hypothalamic neurones, which directly control the secretion of pituitary hormones.

The pituitary gland is made up of two lobes, posterior (neurohypophysis) and anterior (adenohypophysis), the names explaining why removal of the gland is called 'hypophysectomy'. The posterior lobe releases two peptides:

(a) oxytocin, controlling uterine contractions at birth and affecting milk 'let-down';
(b) vasopressin (antidiuretic hormone), stimulating water reabsorption by the kidney tubules.

The anterior lobe synthesizes several hormones, each from a distinct cell type; secretion is largely regulated by local peptide hormones liberated from peptidergic neurones in the hypothalamus. These substances are carried to the pituitary via the hypophyseal portal veins. In turn the hypothalamic peptidergic neurones are affected by higher centres through catecholamine or 5-hydroxytryptamine pathways. In the case of the pituitary hormone prolactin, inhibitory control is exerted not by a peptide but by dopamine carried from the hypothalamus by portal veins.

A complex interrelationship exists between these neurotransmitters, the releasing (or release-inhibiting) hormones, the pituitary hormones and the cells which ultimately respond (many being peripheral endocrine glands which secrete yet more hormones). For instance, negative feedback loops are

Hypothalamic releasing hormones (RHs) or release-inhibiting hormones (RIHs)	Anterior pituitary product	Major function
Corticotrophin RH (CRH)	Corticotrophin (adrenocorticotrophic hormone; ACTH)	Acts on adrenal cortex (e.g. glucocorticoid release)
Gonadotrophin RH (GRH)		
(a) Follicle-stimulating hormone RH (FSHRH)	(a) FSH	Ovum, Graafian follicle growth
(b) Luteinizing hormone RH (LHRH)	(b) LH (In male known as interstitial cell-stimulating hormone; ICSH)	Corpus luteum growth LH and FSH together regulate oestrogen/progesterone secretion
Growth hormone RH (GHRH) Somatostatin (GHRIH)	Growth hormone (somatotrophin)	Regulates bodily growth, directly and by hepatic release of somatomedins
Prolactin RIH (Dopamine; PRIH)	Prolactin	Breast development and milk production
Thyrotrophin RH (TRH)	Thyrotrophin	Synthesis/secretion from thyroid

The anterior pituitary also releases melanocyte-stimulating hormone, which affects skin pigmentation in amphibia but whose functions in man are unknown.

continued on next page

common and the final secretory product from a peripheral endocrine gland may act on hypothalamic neurones to inhibit peptide release (e.g. glucocorticoids from the adrenal gland inhibit corticotrophin releasing hormone, thereby limiting the secretion of corticotrophin from the pituitary). Therefore the effects of drugs on the endocrine systems may be brought about by actions at many different points in these pathways. TTFFF

The anterior lobe (adenohypophysis) of the pituitary gland

1. releases dopamine, which suppresses lactation.
2. has a role in the control of body water by secreting vasopressin (antidiuretic hormone).
3. has been a source of human growth hormone used to treat dwarfism.
4. responds to neuroleptic drugs with a reduction in prolactin secretion.
5. is influenced by peptide releasing-hormones carried in a portal venous system from the hypothalamus.

The hormones of the pituitary gland and their associated releasing hormones from peptidergic neurones of the hypothalamus are all peptides. They range in size from the tripeptide (pyroglutamyl-histidyl-proline) thyrotrophin releasing hormone to molecules with more than 200 amino acids – the gonadotrophic hormones. For several reasons, most of these peptides are unsuitable for therapeutic use (instability, immunogenicity, poor absorption). However, some analogues are available such as **felypressin** (more stable than vasopressin and used as a vasoconstrictor in local anaesthesia) and **tetracosactrin** (a lower molecular weight derivative of corticotrophin (adrenocorticotrophic hormone) with lower immunogenicity). The availability of hormones in pure form in large quantities through genetic engineering may reduce the dangers both of allergic reactions and of viral transmission associated with preparations derived from cadaver tissue.

Growth hormone (somatotrophin) has been used successfully to treat pituitary dwarfism. However, distribution of all human pituitary products ceased in 1985 when some patients given growth hormones several years earlier developed Creutzfeld–Jakob disease (a fatal neurodegenerative condition transmitted by a virus in the pituitary extracts). The clinical usefulness of **growth hormone** produced by genetic engineering has not yet been established. In the future, **growth hormone releasing hormone** may become available as an alternative to growth hormone itself.

The pituitary secretion of prolactin (a peptide structurally similar to growth hormone) is unusual in being under tonic inhibitory control. Cells secreting prolactin possess dopamine (DA) receptors which respond to DA transported by portal veins from the hypothalamus where it is liberated from dopaminergic nerves. Dopamine is considered to be the prolactin release inhibiting hormone (PRIH). These facts explain how some drugs affect prolactin secretion: for instance it is increased by neuroleptic drugs (e.g. some phenothiazines, butyrophenones) which act by blocking DA receptors, or by amine-depleting drugs like **reserpine**; alternatively, agonists like **apomorphine** and **bromocriptine** suppress release by mimicking PRIH. Thus predictable side-effects of neuroleptic drugs include lactation and gynaecomastia.

Hyperprolactinaemia is a condition which may occur, for example, with certain pituitary tumours or as an unwanted drug-induced effect. It may be treated with the dopamine agonist **bromocriptine** which, in cases of pituitary tumours, will relieve the gynaecomastia in males and restore ovulatory menstruation in females. **Bromocriptine** may also be used after childbirth to suppress lactation without causing breast engorgement. FFTFT

MCQ 169

Oral contraceptive preparations

1. of the 'combined' type, contain lower doses of oestrogen than of progestogen.
2. which contain progestogen alone act by suppressing ovulation.
3. increase the risk of thromboembolic disorders about 20-fold.
4. decrease the incidence of ovarian cancer.
5. may predispose women to iron-deficiency anaemia.

During the menstrual cycle, physiological changes occur which prepare the reproductive system for potential pregnancy. Pathological disturbances in the cyclical release and integrated action of female sex hormones may lead to an undesired state of infertility. Alternatively, drugs may be used purposely to disturb the endocrine cycle, thereby acting as contraceptives. Their action may be understood by reference to the factors governing the normal menstrual cycle.

When stimulated by a releasing hormone from the hypothalamus, cells in the anterior pituitary liberate follicle-stimulating hormone (FSH), which causes growth of the ovarian follicles. That follicle containing the ovum which may become fertilized (Graafian follicle) develops more quickly at the expense of the remainder, which degenerate; it begins to secrete oestrogens. Among other actions, oestrogens:

(a) prepare the uterus for implantation of a fertilized ovum (proliferative phase);
(b) reduce the FSH output;
(c) help promote the secretion of luteinizing hormone (LH) from the pituitary;
(d) stimulate the formation of progesterone receptors in target tissues.

Luteinizing hormone acts first to rupture the Graafian follicle, releasing the ovum, and next to cause development of the progesterone-secreting corpus luteum from the follicle. Progesterone further prepares the oestrogen-primed uterus for implantation (secretory phase); it also causes inhibition of release of LH from the pituitary. If implantation fails to occur, progesterone secretion stops, leading to the onset of menstruation.

Oral contraceptive drugs fall into two categories, the first a combination of oestrogen and progestogen, the second progestogen alone. The 'combined pill', taken for 3 weeks and omitted for 1 week, is thought to (a) suppress FSH release (oestrogen component of the pill), so that follicular development is inhibited, and (b) suppress LH release (progestogen component), thereby preventing ovulation. Withdrawal leads to menstruation. A less reliable method of contraception involves progestogen alone, taken every day without a break, which may act to alter the mucus composition (so that sperm survive less well) and possibly to hinder implantation of any ova which become fertilized. However, unlike the combined preparations, progestogen alone may be used after childbirth as lactation is unaffected.

Undesirable effects are more marked with the combined preparation, the

continued on next page

oestrogen component being largely responsible, which is the reason why the oestrogen dose has been lowered (e.g. **ethinyl oestradiol** 50 μg or less). Doses of progestogen (e.g. **norgesterol, norethisterone**) are 5- to 20-fold greater than those of oestrogen although the trend has been to reduce these also. Potentially most serious is the risk of thrombosis, although the advent of low-dose oestrogen pills has reduced its incidence to about three times higher than in women not taking these drugs. The risk of cervical cancer is slightly higher and diabetes may develop in some women. Other unwanted effects like weight gain, jaundice and increased skin pigmentation are associated with the progestogen component. The obvious beneficial effect is a decreased likelihood of unwanted pregnancy; but, in addition, there is a lower risk of uterine and ovarian cancer, a reduction of iron-deficiency anaemia (by about 50%), of certain breast tumours and of premenstrual tension. TFFTF

MCQ 170

Adrenocortical insufficiency may occur

1. in Addison's disease or after prolonged glucocorticoid therapy.
2. in Cushing's syndrome.
3. after administration of **metyrapone**.
4. in phaeochromocytoma.
5. in hypopituitarism.

The adrenal gland is divided into an outer (cortical) layer, which produces both glucocorticoids and mineralocorticoids, and a central medulla, which synthesizes catecholamines. Excessive amounts of adrenaline may arise from an adrenal medullary tumour or from overgrowth of chromaffin tissue elsewhere in the body (called 'phaeochromocytoma'). Excessive sweating and hypertension will result from the high plasma levels of adrenaline and the urinary excretion of vanillylmandelic acid (an adrenaline metabolite) is very high. However, the adrenal cortex is not involved.

Addison's disease is caused by a lack of adrenocortical hormones which occurs when the adrenal cortex is damaged, for example, by an autoimmune process, by carcinoma or by infection. Production of these hormones can also be prevented by drugs. The experimental tool **aminoglutethimide** blocks the production of pregnenolone from cholesterol and so reduces the synthesis of all steroids because this conversion is the first stage in the production of glucocorticoids, mineralocorticoids and sex hormones. **Metyrapone** inhibits the formation of hydrocortisone and corticosterone by blocking at a later stage in the pathway. Since these products normally have a negative feedback effect on the hypothalamus and pituitary, this inhibitory control is lost and corticotrophin (adrenocorticotrophic hormone; ACTH) plasma levels rise. Therefore **metyrapone** can be used diagnostically to check pituitary function and may also be used therapeutically to treat glucocorticoid excess (Cushing's syndrome).

Administration of glucocorticoids activates the feedback mechanism which senses the levels of glucocorticoids in the plasma. The feedback mechanism controls adrenal activity through corticotrophin releasing hormone and hence ACTH. Thus the stimulus to the adrenal to synthesize and release cortical hormones is reduced and, if this persists for several weeks, adrenal atrophy will result. If glucocorticoid therapy is stopped, the atrophied adrenal gland cannot produce adequate amounts of these hormones and adrenocortical insufficiency results. Damage to or poor development of the pituitary also causes low levels of ACTH and a consequential adrenocortical insufficiency.

Lack of glucocorticoids causes nausea, vomiting, loss of appetite, fatigue, reduced heart size and ECG changes, hypotension and hypoglycaemia. **Cortisone** or **hydrocortisone** may be used as replacement therapy.

Lack of mineralocorticoids (principally aldosterone) produces hyponatraemia, hyperkalaemia (low sodium and high potassium respectively), dehydration, hypotension and mental changes. **Fludrocortisone** is usually used as replacement therapy. TFTFT

Mineralocorticoids

1. stimulate sodium reabsorption and cause potassium retention.
2. can cause hypertension.
3. can cause muscle weakness.
4. are secreted in excess in Conn's syndrome.
5. are exemplified by aldosterone and **fludrocortisone**.

Aldosterone is the main naturally occurring mineralocorticoid. Hydrocortisone (cortisol) is also released by the adrenal cortex and accounts for about 25% of total endogenous mineralocorticoid activity. They stimulate the reabsorption from the distal tubule of sodium, in exchange for potassium some of which is therefore lost. Subacute administration of mineralocorticoids leads therefore to hypernatraemia and hypokalaemia. Within a few days, however, sodium balance returns to normal though the hypokalaemia is maintained. The potassium-depleted kidney becomes insensitive to vasopressin (antidiuretic hormone) and an increased urine flow results (a type of nephrogenic diabetes insipidus). The low potassium levels also cause skeletal muscle weakness. The alterations in ion transport are not confined to the kidney and the ionic composition of sweat, saliva and other secretions is also changed.

If the effects of endogenous mineralocorticoids on the kidney are blocked, a diuretic effect is seen. Thus **spironolactone**, an aldosterone antagonist, produces a loss of sodium and water and retention of potassium. It is especially useful in conjunction with thiazide diuretics because it can counteract the excessive potassium loss produced by these agents.

Conn's syndrome, usually produced by a tumour of the zona glomerulosa of the adrenal cortex, involves primary hyperaldosteronism and moderate hypertension. Excessive aldosterone production secondary to other disorders (e.g. cirrhosis of the liver, renal disease) is often accompanied by raised renin and angiotensin levels, which may cause severe hypertension. Renin, secreted within the kidney, splits an inactive decapeptide (angiotensin I) from a plasma globulin precursor. In turn, the decapeptide is converted to the octapeptide angiotensin II, a powerful vasoconstrictor agent which also promotes the formation and release of aldosterone from the adrenal cortex. The resulting hypertension may be treated by drugs such as **captopril** or **enalapril** which block angiotensin converting enzyme.

Aldosterone occurs naturally, but is rarely used in therapy because it must be given parenterally and its action is brief. **Fludrocortisone** is a synthetic corticosteroid which is orally active. Its mineralocorticoid activity occurs in about one-tenth the dose needed for glucocorticoid actions. Nonetheless, it is still more potent a glucocorticoid than hydrocortisone, the major endogenous glucocorticoid. FTTTT

Corticosteroids such as **hydrocortisone**

1. may promote glycogen production.
2. promote sodium retention and potassium loss.
3. interact with membrane-bound steroid receptors.
4. inhibit endogenous glucocorticoid synthesis.
5. have an anti-inflammatory effect.

Naturally occurring adrenocortical hormones like hydrocortisone (cortisol; the major glucocorticoid in man) and corticosterone (the major one in the rat), and synthetic analogues such as **prednisolone**, have two main properties. They exhibit glucocorticoid and mineralocorticoid activities. A major clinical application of glucocorticoids is for an anti-inflammatory effect, in which case **dexamethasone**, **betamethasone** and **triamcinolone**, which possess little mineralocorticoid activity, are preferred. However, significant mineralocorticoid activity occurs with many steroids, including **hydrocortisone**, especially when they are administered therapeutically. The main endogenous mineralocorticoid in man is aldosterone, which promotes sodium reabsorption and potassium excretion, leading respectively to increased blood pressure and muscle weakness.

There is a diurnal rhythm in the production of endogenous glucocorticoids (maximum at 06.00 h; minimum at 21.00 h). Moreover, stress causes corticotrophin (adrenocorticotrophic hormone; ACTH) to be liberated from the anterior pituitary (adenohypophysis) and thereby stimulates steroid synthesis. Corticotrophin releasing hormone and ACTH release are also under negative feedback control from the plasma levels of glucocorticoids.

The biological effects of glucocorticoids are initiated when the steroid crosses the cell membrane and combines with a receptor in the cytosol of the cell. The receptor–steroid complex is then translocated to the nucleus, RNA polymerases are activated and transcription of specific messenger RNA is initiated. Ribosomal enzyme synthesis is thus stimulated.

Glucocorticoids cause increased gluconeogenesis (utilizing peptides and amino acids from skeletal muscle, hence muscle weakness on prolonged therapy) and the resulting glucose is stored as glycogen. Lipolysis in response to adrenaline, growth hormone or glucagon can only occur if glucocorticoids are present. The cardiovascular system is also affected and low blood pressure and reduced cardiac force are produced if levels of glucocorticoids are low. Adrenaline synthesis in the adrenal medulla is affected as phenylethanolamine *N*-methyltransferase is induced when high concentrations of cortical hormones reach the adjacent medulla in its blood supply. Central nervous system effects include euphoria, restlessness and increased motor activity. Whenever glucocorticoids are used therapeutically, large amounts are given, which may cause a change in the distribution of fat in the body and give rise to 'moon-face' or, in extreme cases, to 'buffalo-hump'. TTFTT

The thyroid gland

1. is located between the larynx and the vertebral column.
2. actively takes up **iodide** from the plasma in order to iodinate tyramine.
3. may produce inadequate amounts of thyroid hormones, giving rise to Graves' disease (myxoedema in adults or cretinism in children).
4. may be partly removed by surgery as a treatment for thyrotoxicosis.
5. is involved in the control of growth.

The thyroid gland is located in the neck, *ventral* to the trachea, not between it and the spine. The gland accumulates iodide from the plasma and iodinates tyrosine, which is incorporated in pre-formed thyroglobulin (a glycoprotein containing some 100 tyrosine residues). Pairs of mono- and di-iodotyrosine residues are linked to form tri-iodothyronine (T_3) and tetra-iodothyronine (thyroxine; T_4). They remain incorporated in the thyroglobulin molecule until their release is triggered. Tri-iodothyronine is more potent than thyroxine and, although present in lower concentrations in plasma, is less protein-bound. Both materials thus contribute to the overall effect.

Underproduction of thyroid hormones (hypothyroidism) leads to myxoedema in adults (low metabolic rate, bradycardia, mental and physical slowing) and to cretinism in children (mental retardation and dwarfism). Dwarfism is produced since thyroid hormones increase the output of growth hormone (somatotrophin). Iodide deficiency can also be responsible for hypothyroidism and can lead to excessive growth of the gland and to goitre, the classical swelling of the neck. In goitre, the low thyroid hormone levels fail to suppress the release of thyroid-stimulating hormone (TSH). The excess TSH stimulates thyroid activity and causes the gland to hypertrophy (in an attempt to produce sufficient hormones). To prevent such symptoms, **iodide** is routinely added to table salt (iodized salt).

Overproduction of thyroid hormones (hyperthyroidism; thyrotoxicosis; Graves' disease) produces a high metabolic rate, sweating, tremor, weight loss and increased appetite. These symptoms may be due to the presence of a long-acting thyroid-stimulating substance (LATS) from extrathyroid sources.

In both conditions diagnosis is by symptomatology and by measuring the uptake of **iodine-131** (^{131}I) using the γ-emissions from this β- and γ-radionuclide (half-life 8 days). Therapy of *hypo*thyroidism is hormone replacement. Therapy of *hyper*thyroidism is by surgical removal of part of the gland, by part destruction using the β-emission from much larger doses of ^{131}I than are used in diagnosis, or with antithyroid drugs. FFFTT

MCQ 174

Of the drugs which may be used in the management of hyperthyroidism

1. **perchlorate** and **thiocyanate** inhibit iodide uptake into the thyroid gland.
2. **carbimazole** and **methimazole** reduce the synthesis of tri-iodothyronine and thyroxine.
3. **methyl-** and **iodo-thiouracil** prevent the formation of mono-iodo-thyronine.
4. *p*-**aminosalicylic acid** reduces iodide uptake by the thyroid.
5. **propranolol** counteracts the symptoms and does not correct the hormonal defect.

Hyperthyroidism may be controlled by drugs of two major groups. One type reduces the uptake of iodide by the gland (**perchlorate, thiocyanate** and **fluoroborate**). The other type (**carbimazole, methimazole, methyl-** and **iodo-thiouracil**) reduces the synthesis of tri- (T_3) and tetra-iodothyronine (thyroxine; T_4). Iodination of the tyrosine residues to form mono- and di-iodothyronine is relatively unaffected, but the linkage of these materials to form tri- and tetra-iodothyronine is reduced. Some undesirable effects occur with these antithyroid drugs, for example rashes, headaches, gastrointestinal upsets and, occasionally, serious blood dyscrasias.

Thiocyanate and **fluoroborate** are largely obsolete now and **perchlorate** is used only occasionally. Other forms of therapy are not entirely without risk. Surgery may damage the adjacent parathyroid glands with consequential changes in calcium metabolism and also carries the usual risks attendant on general anaesthesia. **Iodine-131** can lead to slowly developing hypothyroidism.

p-**Aminosalicylic acid** (an antitubercular drug) does not affect iodide uptake but on long-term administration produces a hypothyroid syndrome in about 20% of patients. **Propranolol** does not affect the thyroid directly but is used in the treatment of hyperthyroidism to combat the tremor, tachycardia and generalized symptoms of sympathetic overactivity.

Iodide itself can produce an antithyroid effect in large doses (6 mg per day as opposed to the 0.2 mg dietary requirement). The gland shrinks and becomes less vascular after about 15 days therapy. This effect is often short-lived, however and the hyperthyroidism may return more severely than was originally the case. For this reason **iodide** treatment is used only before surgery to reduce the vascularity of the gland and make the surgical procedure somewhat easier. TTFFT

Insulin

1. is released from pancreatic α-cells by α-adrenoceptor agonists.
2. stimulates gluconeogenesis and lipolysis.
3. produces its peak effect in about 3 h but has a plasma half-life of a few minutes.
4. from man and pig is identical in amino acid composition.
5. causes effects which are counteracted by glucagon.

The polypeptide hormone insulin (51 amino acids in chains A and B linked by two sulphide bonds) is released by pancreatic β-cells. It is formed by cleavage of its precursor, pro-insulin and stored until required. Other products are released from different pancreatic cells (e.g. glucagon, somatostatin). The major stimulus for insulin release is an increase in blood glucose concentration, the β-cells responding both to absolute concentration and to the rate of change. Insulin secretion is stimulated by several hormones and by agonists at β_2-adrenoceptors (but is inhibited by α-adrenoceptor agonists).

Insulin has several important metabolic effects, which include:

(a) increased glucose uptake into many tissues, after which the glucose may contribute to raised biosynthesis of glycogen, glycerol, fatty acids (depending on cell type);

(b) elevated amino acid uptake and protein synthesis, especially in muscle cells;

(c) decreases in glycogenolysis and gluconeogenesis (thereby decreasing glucose release particularly from the liver) and in adipocytic lipolysis.

Insulin belongs to a family of polypeptides, several of which contribute to insulin-like activity in plasma. Furthermore, the structure of insulin differs between species, porcine being closest to human insulin with alanine substituting for threonine in position 30. For therapeutic purposes, **insulin** may be obtained from pigs or cattle, but '**human insulin**' can now be produced in large quantities by recombinant DNA technology using bacteria such as *Escherichia coli*.

It is important that mechanisms exist to regulate plasma levels of nutrients since the demand for them varies (e.g. increases during exercise) and their supply is intermittent (e.g. higher at meal times). Thus, after feeding, excess blood glucose will be taken into cells for storage as glycogen or fat which, in turn, can be mobilized during fasting or by demands such as exercise. The major effect of insulin to lower blood glucose levels is counteracted by several hormones (principally glucagon from pancreatic α-cells, but also adrenaline, glucocorticoids and growth hormone) which are liberated during episodes of hypoglycaemia.

Insulin has a rapid onset of effect (1–2 min) but, since the peak effect occurs after 2–4 h whilst its plasma half-life is a few minutes only, there must be major tissue binding and prolonged intracellular changes. It is known that an insulin receptor exists on the surface of its target cells; the receptor has

continued on next page 213

been purified and characterized. Binding of insulin induces phosphorylation of the receptor and the complex is internalized, leading to a cascade of further phosphorylation reactions within the cell as well as to the production of a novel second messenger (inositol phosphate glycan). The insulin receptor is recycled and intracellular insulin is degraded. Many changes in enzyme activity and several reaction products have been noted during cellular stimulation by insulin, although their relationship to the functional responses is not yet well understood. FFTFT

Diabetes mellitus

1. of the 'juvenile-onset' type involves a profound loss of pancreatic β-cells.
2. of the 'late-onset' type is associated with lack of vasopressin (antidiuretic hormone).
3. of both types may require **insulin** therapy.
4. is associated with long-term complications of vascular lesions and neuropathies.
5. of both types responds to treatment with oral hypoglycaemic agents.

Diabetes *insipidus* is a rare condition due to lack of vasopressin (antidiuretic hormone) and should not be confused with diabetes mellitus, which is associated with a low insulin activity. Patients with untreated diabetes mellitus are:

(a) hyperglycaemic (tissues cannot use glucose or store glycogen);
(b) glycosuric (excess glucose appears in the urine);
(c) polyuric and polydipsic (urinary glucose causes diuresis, which stimulates fluid intake);
(d) ketotic (from increased lipolysis).

Long-term diabetic patients are at risk from vascular lesions, particularly in the eye and kidney, and demyelinating neuropathies.

The disorder presents in two forms: (a) juvenile-onset (insulin dependent diabetes mellitus; IDDM) and (b) late-onset (non-insulin dependent diabetes mellitus; NIDDM). In the case of IDDM, there is an extensive loss of pancreatic β-cells, which leads to a virtual lack of plasma insulin and a failure to respond to the stimulus of hyperglycaemia. In many patients, antibodies to the β-cells are found in the plasma, though in some cases viral damage to the cells is suspected. The major, logical treatment of IDDM is **insulin**. By contrast, NIDDM is gradual in onset and is not associated with major losses of β-cells; however, there may be insensitivity of target cells to insulin or defects in glucose-sensing by the β-cells. The presence of antibodies to the β-cells is rare. Since patients suffering NIDDM are often overweight, diet alone may suffice although **insulin** or oral hypoglycaemic drug therapy may be needed.

Insulin, being a large polypeptide, cannot be given orally and is therefore given by self-injection (or by an automatic infusor) subcutaneously. In order to avoid hypoglycaemia and ketoacidosis, individual dosing regimes are necessary and, towards this end, three categories of preparations are available: fast-, intermediate- or slow-acting. Fast-acting soluble **insulins** are in buffered neutral solutions which can be given i.v. in emergencies. The slower-acting ones, whose effects may last for up to 36 h from a single injection, are preparations of large crystals of **zinc–insulin** or of **insulin** bound to **protamine**, which dissolve slowly; alterations to the crystal size will alter the rate of absorption. The **zinc–insulin** suspensions which are available in each of the categories are appropriately termed semilente, lente and

continued on next page

ultralente to indicate their respectively slower rates of dissolution. The dose regimen for a particular patient may require adjustment according to his or her physical state, for example exercise, infections, pregnancy. Patients are better able to control their condition with the advent of home testing kits to measure blood or urinary glucose. Nonetheless, complications may occur if **insulin** resistance develops. There is evidence that the surging changes in blood glucose levels which still occur in diabetic patients treated with **insulin** contribute to the vascular lesions. Trials are continuing with implanted devices which monitor glucose concentration and deliver **insulin** accordingly. If the technique proves successful and reliable, the incidence of pathological changes in chronic diabetes might become lower.

Since oral hypoglycaemic drugs require functional pancreatic β-cells (from which they promote insulin release), they are not used to treat IDDM. TFTTF

In the pancreatectomized animal the rise in blood glucose seen after a meal would be significantly reduced by the administration of

1. glucagon.
2. adrenaline.
3. chlorpropamide.
4. metformin.
5. glibenclamide.

Removal of the pancreas eliminates not only its exocrine contribution to digestion but also the source of insulin and glucagon and one of the sources of somatostatin (found also in the CNS and gastrointestinal tract). The hyperglycaemia after a meal is, therefore, unopposed because insulin can no longer be released no matter what the stimulus.

Glucagon is one of several factors besides glucose which cause insulin release, but this is impossible in a pancreatectomized animal. On its target tissues, **glucagon** produces effects opposite from insulin. By stimulating adenylate cyclase, it raises intracellular cyclic AMP concentrations and (e.g. in liver cells) the consequent activation of a protein kinase leads to a cascade of reactions culminating in glycogenolysis and gluconeogenesis. Therefore blood glucose is likely to rise further and the hyperglycaemia following a meal would not be counteracted. A rise in cyclic AMP, with similar consequences, would occur with **adrenaline**, which activates adenylate cyclase by stimulating β-adrenoceptors. In an intact animal the effect of adrenaline would be complex since not only would the pancreas already be responding to changes in blood glucose but also the release of insulin is (a) decreased by α-adrenoceptor agonists and (b) increased by stimulation of β-adrenoceptors on the pancreatic β-cells.

Two major chemical groups of oral hypoglycaemic agents exist: sulphonylureas and biguanides. Although the mechanisms of action are not completely understood, these drugs are never used in the treatment of 'juvenile-onset' diabetes mellitus (insulin dependent diabetes mellitus; IDDM) but only in the 'late-onset' type where functional β-cells exist in large numbers (non-insulin dependent diabetes mellitus; NIDDM). The sulphonylureas (which include **chlorpropamide, tolbutamide, glibenclamide, glymidine**) are entirely dependent on the presence of insulin for their effect and they increase insulin release as well as possibly altering its binding or metabolism. Therefore they will be ineffective in the pancreatectomized animal. When used therapeutically, they may cause skin rashes and gastrointestinal disturbances though severe side-effects seldom occur. Nonetheless, a satisfactory control of blood glucose is achieved with drugs of this type in fewer than one-third of NIDDM patients undergoing prolonged treatment.

Of the biguanides, **metformin** is the only agent used therapeutically. Its precise mode of action is unknown. Although experiments were reported in which **phenformin** (another biguanide) caused a reduction in blood glucose levels in pancreatectomized dogs, these findings have not been confirmed using **metformin** in pancreatectomized dogs or humans. After

continued on next page

subtotal pancreatectomy in humans, the resulting diabetes has been controlled by **metformin** alone. Thus there is little evidence to suggest that **metformin** would be effective in the experiment outlined above. In clinical use **metformin** may take several weeks for its action to become established. It has a variety of undesirable effects including nausea, vomiting, loss of appetite and reduced vitamin B_{12} and folate levels. Occasionally a large and potentially fatal increase occurs in plasma levels of lactic acid. FFFFF

Chemotherapy of Microorganisms

MCQ 178

Antibacterial agents

1. show selective toxicity.
2. may act by inhibiting cell wall synthesis, as do cephalosporins.
3. of the polymixin group inhibit protein synthesis in bacterial and mammalian cells.
4. are classified as antibiotics when they are active *in vivo*.
5. of the sulphonamide group are bacteriostatic because they interfere with nucleic acid synthesis.

Many textbooks use the term 'antibiotic' specifically to describe those antibacterial drugs which are naturally occurring substances (products of moulds, fungi and bacteria themselves), thereby distinguishing them from purely synthetic drugs. This distinction seems to have little point and we will use the term 'antibacterial' throughout.

More lives have been saved this century by antibacterials than by any other class of drug. These agents exhibit selective toxicity, i.e. they inhibit the growth of or kill bacteria at levels which produce few adverse effects on mammalian cells. This selectivity is due to differences between mammalian and bacterial cells which may be exemplified as follows:

Bacterial cells, unlike mammalian cells, possess a rigid cell wall to contain the high osmotic pressure. Drugs like **penicillin** and cephalosporins which weaken the cell wall allow osmotic forces to disrupt the cell and are bactericidal.

Gram-negative bacterial cell membranes are rich in phosphatidyl ethanolamine, which binds strongly to antibacterials of the polymixin group. These drugs act like detergents to damage the plasma membrane and allow leakage of vital materials from the cell.

All living cells synthesize proteins in a fundamentally similar way. Ribosomes bind with a strand of messenger RNA (mRNA) coded for a particular protein, several ribosomes being simultaneously attached like beads along the strand (polysomes). The correct amino acids are then carried to the ribosomes by transfer RNA (tRNA) and linked progressively to form polypeptide chains and, eventually, the protein for which the mRNA was coded. The nature of the subunits which form the ribosomes varies in different types of organism and this variation permits drugs like **tetracycline** and **erythromycin** to affect ribosome function in one species but not another.

Folic acid is an essential intermediate in the synthesis of DNA. Mammalian cells use dietary **folic acid** but most bacteria synthesize their own supply from *p*-aminobenzoic acid (PABA). Sulphonamides compete with PABA for the enzyme which incorporates PABA into folic acid. **Trimethoprim** blocks the production of tetrahydrofolate from folic acid at an intermediate stage by inhibiting dihydrofolate reductase. This reaction takes place in bacteria *and* in mammalian cells but the drug is much more effective against the bacterial (and plasmodial) enzymes. TTFFT

The penicillins are antibacterial drugs

1. that must be administered with other drugs to exert a bactericidal effect.
2. which act to disrupt bacterial cell walls by inhibiting the transpeptidase enzymes which bring about cross-linking.
3. some of which (e.g. **cloxacillin**) are resistant to hydrolysis both by β-lactamase and gastric acid.
4. which have thiazolidine and β-lactam rings, both of which may be cleaved by β-lactamase.
5. some of which (e.g. **ampicillin**) are effective orally.

The bactericidal effects of the mould *Penicillium notatum* were discovered by Fleming in 1928, but more than a decade passed before the full therapeutic potential of **penicillin** was realized through the efforts of Florey and Chain. The original **penicillin** was a mixture of compounds but the individual components can be produced by altering the composition of the medium on which the mould is grown. Nowadays many semisynthetic penicillins are available which overcome the limitations of the earliest penicillin (**benzylpenicillin**).

All penicillins possess a thiazolidine ring attached to a β-lactam ring which has a free amino group. A variety of other groups can be attached at this point to give various semisynthetic penicillins which have different properties. **Benzylpenicillin** has the highest activity against Gram-positive bacteria but is readily hydrolysed by β-lactamase and gastric acid. **Amoxicillin** and **ampicillin** have greater activity than **benzylpenicillin** against Gram-negative organisms (i.e. a broader spectrum), are resistant to gastric acid but are still susceptible to β-lactamase. **Oxacillin** and **cloxacillin** are acid-stable and resistant to hydrolysis by β-lactamase. These are the drugs of choice against β-lactamase-producing staphylococci, but would not be used against organisms sensitive to **benzylpenicillin**, which is both cheap and effective. It should be noted that all bacteria produce at least one β-lactamase directed by chromosomal DNA. Additional β-lactamases may be synthesized through transferred DNA, for example via plasmids. The many enzymes in this family vary greatly in activity and substrate specificity and some bacterial species produce types for which penicillins are poor substrates. **Clavulanic acid** is a 'suicide' inhibitor of β-lactamase and may be used in combination with **amoxicillin** against strains of staphylococci or gonococci which would otherwise hydrolyse the penicillin.

All these penicillins are bactericidal as long as bacteria are growing; metabolically inactive cells are unaffected. The protective bacterial cell wall is composed of elongated carbohydrate strands made up of alternating N-acetylmuramic acid and N-acetylglucosamine molecules which are cross-linked by glycine chains to form peptidoglycan. This cross-linking is initiated by a transpeptidase which is inhibited by **penicillin**. Without the cross-linking the cell wall is weakened and can no longer resist the high internal osmotic pressure. Water, therefore, flows into the cell, which expands and finally ruptures. FTTFT

Cephalosporins

1. possess a β-lactam ring and can therefore be hydrolysed by any β-lactamase.
2. have a broader spectrum of action than **penicillin** and are active against more types of Gram-negative bacteria.
3. are bactericidal since they inhibit transpeptidase and prevent cross-linking in bacterial cell walls.
4. are immunologically cross-reactive with penicillins and should never be used in patients allergic to **penicillin**.
5. are unstable in acid and can be given only intramuscularly or intravenously.

Cephalosporin antibacterials resemble the penicillins. Their mode of action is identical, both groups inhibiting transpeptidase, thereby preventing peptidoglycan cross-linking in the bacterial cell wall. Like penicillins, they possess a β-lactam ring with an attached amino group. Since a wide variety of other groups can be linked to an amino group, a wide range of semisynthetic derivatives are available. Cephalosporins have a broad spectrum of activity against Gram-negative and Gram-positive organisms, including penicillin-resistant staphylococci. The possession of a β-lactam ring means that cephalosporins may be hydrolysed by some β-lactamases. All bacteria produce a β-lactamase, which differs between genus, species and subspecies of organism, whose synthesis is directed by chromosomal DNA. Moreover, additional β-lactamases may be produced as a result of transferred DNA, for example transposon- or plasmid-borne. Some β-lactamases hydrolyse penicillins rapidly, some hydrolyse cephalosporins at a greater rate than penicillins, while others exist for which most β-lactams are poor substrates. The terms 'penicillinase' and 'cephalosporinase' are no longer recognized by the Commission for Enzyme Nomenclature.

Most cephalosporins are hydrolysed by gastric acid and poorly absorbed from the gut. They must, therefore, be given i.m., a painful process, or i.v. Some newer derivatives (**cephalexin** and **cephadrine**) are, however, orally effective and are used mainly for infections of the respiratory or urinary tract.

The major unwanted effect of penicillins is an acute allergic reaction which may be severe enough to cause death. About one person in 50 000 receiving **penicillin** is likely to die from an allergic reaction, but this is a small number compared with those saved by the drug. Some immunological sensitization occurs in 2–10% of patients exposed to **penicillin**. Sensitization can occur without the patients' knowledge, for example by drinking milk from cows which have received **penicillin**. Most penicillins are cross-sensitizing and cross-reacting, the antigenic determinants being degradation products, particularly penicilloic acid linked to a protein. Cephalosporins are often substituted for penicillins in allergic patients, though up to 10% of allergic patients may show cross-allergy between the groups. Cephalosporins can also, of course, give rise to allergy in their own right. FTTFF

Chloramphenicol *and tetracyclines*

1. are broad-spectrum antibacterials originally discovered in strains of *Streptomyces*.
2. both produce only minor side-effects and are used extensively.
3. both can produce the 'grey baby syndrome' through inadequate glucuronidation.
4. prevent bacterial protein synthesis by attaching to the 30 s ribosomal subunit.
5. are bacteriostatic and bind reversibly to intracellular sites.

Chloramphenicol and the earlier tetracyclines were isolated in the late 1940s from different strains of *Streptomyces*. A considerable number of tetracyclines now exist, with a bewildering variety of trade names (many of which terminate in '-mycin'). All have a broad spectrum of activity and are bacteriostatic. Most are resistant to gastric acid and are absorbed from the gastrointestinal tract.

Chloramphenicol, nowadays wholly synthetic, shares many properties with the tetracyclines and also blocks bacterial protein synthesis but is less frequently used clinically because, occasionally, a fatal aplastic anaemia may develop due to depression of the bone marrow. **Chloramphenicol** is the drug of choice in typhoid and paratyphoid fever, for meningitis (because it penetrates the blood–brain barrier readily) and for pneumonias where the organisms are resistant to other drugs. It is occasionally given topically in the treatment of eye infections. Neonates lack the mechanism for glucuronide formation which would normally detoxify **chloramphenicol**, hence the 'grey baby syndrome' (vomiting, hypothermia, grey colour, collapse) due to excessively high **chloramphenicol** plasma levels. These unwanted effects are not seen with tetracyclines, which have a broad spectrum of action and are used extensively for mixed respiratory tract infections, pneumonias and penicillin-resistant gonococci.

Bacterial protein synthesis occurs as follows. Ribosomal subunits (30 s and 50 s) become attached to the end of a messenger RNA (mRNA) strand. An amino acid is transferred by transfer RNA (tRNA) to the ribosome, which then moves along the mRNA strand. The next amino acid is carried in by tRNA and becomes bound to the first to form a dipeptide. The whole process is repeated over and over again to produce a copy of the protein coded by the mRNA strand.

Tetracyclines (e.g. **chlortetracycline**, **oxytetracycline**) bind to a particular site on the 30 s ribosomal subunit, prevent access to tRNA and its amino acid and thus stop the peptide chain from growing. **Chloramphenicol** binds instead to the 50 s subunit, which is hindered from attaching to the mRNA. Both the drugs bind reversibly and plasma concentrations must, therefore, be maintained at effective levels for a long enough time for the host's defence mechanisms to eliminate the bacteria. TFFFT

MCQ 182

Aminoglycoside antibacterials

1. are typified by **Aureomycin** and **Terramycin**.
2. inhibit bacterial protein synthesis and are bactericidal.
3. such as **streptomycin** cause misreading of the genetic code and permit the insertion of incorrect amino acids in the peptide chain.
4. cause liver damage.
5. damage the auditory nerve (cranial nerve VIII), causing vestibular or auditory dysfunction.

Many drugs which act by inhibiting bacterial protein synthesis are bacteriostatic. However, the aminoglycosides (e.g. **streptomycin**) are bactericidal because they have a multiplicity of actions. The majority of aminoglycosides (e.g. **kanamycin, neomycin**) are naturally occurring substances and are (like tetracyclines) isolated from various strains of *Streptomyces*. Some (e.g. **gentamicin**) are obtained from different organisms. **Aureomycin** and **Terramycin** are proprietary names for **chlortetracycline** and **oxytetracycline** respectively and are not aminoglycosides.

The mode of action of **streptomycin** is probably best known and differs little from the others in the group. It first attaches to a specific receptor protein on the 30 s subunit of the bacterial ribosome. This binding may prevent the formation of the 'initiation complex' (messenger RNA + transfer RNA + amino acid) with which peptide formation begins. In higher concentrations, **streptomycin** causes misreading of the genetic code by permitting the attachment of an incorrect amino acid to the growing peptide. This could eventually result in a non-functional protein in which several amino acids have been replaced. Finally, binding of aminoglycosides to the 30 s subunit often results in the disintegration of polysomes (the several ribosomes attached to any complete strand of messenger RNA) to form 'monosomes' which are unable to participate in protein synthesis. These several actions occur more or less simultaneously and usually cause cell death.

Aminoglycosides are very polar compounds, poorly absorbed from the gut and therefore usually given i.m. or i.v. Although many Gram-positive and Gram-negative organisms are susceptible to aminoglycosides, the drugs are used sparingly because of adverse reactions. **Streptomycin** is used in bubonic plague (in conjunction with tetracylines) and in tuberculosis. **Kanamycin** is used in staphylococcal skin infections and to reduce gut flora. **Gentamicin** is used against severe infections with Gram-positive organisms such as *Pseudomonas* and *Proteus*.

All aminoglycosides are ototoxic, capable of damaging the auditory nerve (cranial nerve VIII). **Gentamicin** and **streptomycin** predominantly affect vestibular function and hence balance; **kanamycin** and **neomycin** are more likely to affect hearing. None of these drugs has been reported to cause liver damage although **neomycin** may increase the faecal excretion of bile acids, probably by decreasing their intestinal reabsorption. However, all are nephrotoxic and should be used with extreme care in patients with renal failure. Impaired kidney function leads to high plasma levels of drugs, increasing the risk of severe unwanted effects. In addition, the nephrotoxic action may damage the kidney further. FTTFT

The sulphonamide drugs

1. are wholly synthetic and are not produced by living organisms.
2. vary in duration of action, the short-acting ones being favoured for urinary tract infections.
3. are all potentially nephrotoxic because of low water solubility and the risk of crystalluria.
4. include **sulphasalazine**, which is used as a second-in-line antiarthritic drug.
5. may be used prior to surgery to reduce bacterial populations in the gut, provided the drugs are not absorbed from the intestine.

The first clinically successful antibacterial drugs were sulphonamides. **Sulphanilamide** was synthesized in 1908 but 25 years elapsed before its clinical effectiveness was demonstrated. About 20 sulphonamides have been used extensively and they are grouped according to their lipid solubilities (reflecting ease of absorption from the gut) and their duration of action (dependent on binding to plasma proteins, speed of renal excretion and rate of absorption).

Phthalylsulphathiazole is an almost insoluble compound. It is not absorbed from the gut and is used principally to reduce the bacterial population of the gut in patients about to undergo intestinal surgery.

Sulphamethizole is short-acting, soluble, poorly bound to plasma proteins and little is biotransformed to the toxic, less soluble acetyl derivative. It is rapidly excreted by the kidney, levels in the tubules are high and the drug is used for urinary tract infections.

Poorly soluble sulphonamides (and the even less soluble acetyl derivatives produced by biotransformation) may crystallize in the renal tubules, causing pain, haematuria and even anuria. Maintenance of a good flow of alkaline urine minimizes the risk of crystalluria as does use of the more soluble sulphonamides.

Long-acting sulphonamides (**sulphadimethoxine** and **sulphasalazine**) are highly (>80%) bound to plasma proteins and are reabsorbed from the kidney tubules. **Sulphadimethoxine** is unusual in that most is excreted as the glucuronide. They are used against some staphylococcal infections and **sulphasalazine** is used to treat ulcerative colitis. Increasingly, **sulphasalazine** is being used to treat rheumatoid arthritis. In cases where symptoms of painful polyarthritis are inadequately controlled by first-line drugs (non-steroidal anti-inflammatory agents), the use of second-line 'disease-modifying' agents may be helpful. **Sulphasalazine** has the most favourable risk : benefit ratio among drugs in this group and may therefore be preferred by some physicians. TTFFT

MCQ 184

The synthesis of nucleic acids

1. requires that folic acid is converted into tetrahydrofolate prior to incorporation of thymidine into DNA.
2. is inhibited in all cells if dihydrofolate reductase is blocked.
3. in many bacterial cells can be prevented by sulphonamides because they compete with *p*-aminobenzoic acid for incorporation into folic acid.
4. may be prevented by **trimethoprim**, which stops the transport of folate into cells.
5. is not essential in those bacteria which are resistant to sulphonamides.

Sulphonamides differ quantitatively but all share the same mechanism of antibacterial action. They are bacteriostatic and inhibit the growth of Gram-positive and Gram-negative organisms, but are ineffective against tuberculosis, typhoid or paratyphoid. Sulphonamides prevent nucleic acid synthesis; this action inhibits bacterial multiplication and allows natural body defences to cope with the infection.

In 1940, Woods and Fildes independently provided the basis for an understanding of how sulphonamides work. All cells convert folic acid to dihydrofolate and then to tetrahydrofolate, which is used in the process of incorporating thymidine into DNA. Most bacteria synthesize their own supply of folate from pteridine, glutamic acid and *p*-aminobenzoic acid (PABA). Mammalian cells lack the enzymes for its synthesis but they take up and use **folic acid** from the diet. Because of its close structural similarity to PABA, the sulphonamide competes for dihydropteroate synthetase and a non-functional analogue of folic acid is produced in which the sulphonamide replaces PABA. Like all competitive inhibitions, the effect is dependent on the relative concentrations of the competing substances and the block can be overcome by adding PABA. Some organisms resistant to sulphonamides have a higher than normal PABA content.

Trimethoprim and the sulphonamide **sulphamethoxazole** are often combined (**Co-trimoxazole**) because they act on different steps in the PABA–folate–tetrahydrofolate–protein pathway and their effects are synergistic. **Trimethoprim** also stops tetrahydrofolate formation but by inhibiting dihydrofolate reductase. This step in nucleic acid synthesis also occurs in mammalian cells, but **trimethoprim** is not harmful to man since it is about 50 000 times more effective on the bacterial enzyme than on human dihydrofolate reductase. While sulphonamides are only bacteriostatic (the natural body defences then killing the bacteria), the combined preparation **Co-trimoxazole** is bactericidal, which often confers an advantage. TTTFF

The origins of drug resistance in bacteria

1. are entirely based on genetic changes.
2. may depend on either chromosomal or extrachromosomal DNA pools.
3. include the transfer of plasmids from one bacterial cell to another by viruses.
4. may involve conjugation of cells and consequent transfer of chromosomal DNA.
5. may involve plasmids which carry genes encoding for multiple drug resistance.

Drug resistance in microorganisms originates in many ways. It can occur when organisms become dormant, since most antibacterials work only on growing cells. Some mycobacteria can remain dormant for years, restrained from replicating by the host's defence mechanisms. If the immunosuppressive corticosteroid drugs are given, then multiplication may start, but the organisms ought to be as susceptible to drugs as the original colony since no genetic change has taken place.

Most types of resistance, however, have a genetic origin. One type develops through spontaneous mutation within the chromosomes of the bacteria which leads to changes in the structure of target proteins. Often the change will occur at a critical point such as the site where **streptomycin** binds to the 30 s subunit of the ribosome. The mutant organism, therefore, no longer binds **streptomycin** and is resistant. Therapy with **streptomycin** leads to selective growth of the resistant organisms at the expense of non-resistant ones, which die.

Bacteria carry extra, non-chromosomal DNA in the form of intracellular particles called plasmids. This DNA also contains genetic information and enables the cells to make proteins other than those coded in the chromosomal DNA. Plasmids often carry information which enables bacteria to synthesize enzymes that can destroy antibacterial drugs (β-lactamases, for example) and therefore cause resistance.

Transfer of genetic material (plasmid and chromosomal) can occur between bacterial cells and so the property of drug resistance can be passed on. These transfers may be by

(a) *transduction* (plasmid carried by a virus from one bacteria to another);
(b) *translocation* (the exchange of short DNA sequences between plasmid and chromosome);
(c) *conjugation* (where DNA is transferred during the mating process and may carry resistance factors to an otherwise susceptible cell).

Once resistance has developed to one member of a group of antibacterial drugs, the bacteria are often cross-resistant to other drugs from the same group. FTTTT

MCQ 186

Bacteria may become resistant to

1. penicillins by developing a changed membrane permeability.
2. cephalosporins by producing a β-lactamase enzyme.
3. sulphonamides because the bacteria develop an uptake process for *p*-aminobenzoic acid.
4. **streptomycin** when they adopt an alternative pathway of protein synthesis which no longer requires the 30 s ribosome.
5. aminoglycosides by adapting to an existence where they no longer require a cell wall.

Microorganisms which are resistant to particular antibacterial drugs cause great concern. Most types of resistance are of genetic origin but the mechanisms involved are diverse.

Many antibacterial drugs work by inhibiting a crucial enzyme; others act as false precursors in a biosynthetic process eventually yielding a non-functional product. Resistance to these types of antibacterial drug could occur if microorganisms developed an alternative biosynthetic pathway. Sulphonamide resistance can be caused by the production of dihydropteroate synthetase which has a much higher affinity for *p*-aminobenzoic acid than for the sulphonamide. Alternatively, some bacteria utilize external **folic acid** (as do mammalian cells) and have, therefore, circumvented the need to synthesize their own folic acid. Hence they lack the process on which suphonamides act.

There is a large family of β-lactamase enzymes which vary greatly in their substrate specificity and degree of activity in hydrolysing β-lactam molecules. Bacteria may synthesize additional β-lactamases if they take in appropriately coded DNA, for example transferred by plasmids. Resistance can occur when bacteria produce β-lactamases which hydrolyse, for example, **benzylpenicillin**. However, some penicillins are hydrolysed less readily (e.g. **oxacillin**) and may therefore be effective in organisms which have become resistant to the more easily hydrolysed penicillins.

Some types of antibacterial agent have to penetrate the cell membrane to work. For example, many tetracyclines enter cells by an active transport process as do many aminoglycosides. Resistance can develop in some bacteria by an acquired change in membrane permeability or in the active uptake processes which transport the antibacterial drugs into the cell.

Another common mechanism by which bacteria develop resistance is by an alteration in the drug target site (receptor). In the case of **streptomycin** its binding site on the 30 s ribosomal subunit can be altered, or, in the case of **erythromycin**, the binding site on the 50 s subunit. These alterations cause failure of binding of the antibacterial agent and hence resistance will have developed. FTFFF

Antimalarial drugs

1. like **quinine** and **chloroquine** act by killing the erythrocytic schizonts.
2. can be classifed by chemical structure and include aminoquinolines and biguanides.
3. include **primaquine**, a folate antagonist which is synergistic with **trimethoprim**.
4. cannot be used in patients with sickle cell anaemia.
5. like **proguanil** and **pyrimethamine** act principally as sporonticides.

Malaria is caused by a protozoal parasite, *Plasmodium*, four species of which infect man. *Plasmodium* enters the bloodstream as a sporozoite when a human is bitten by an infected female mosquito. It enters the liver cell, where it becomes a schizont which then divides into daughter merozoites. These are liberated into the blood as the liver cell ruptures. Some merozoites may reinfect other liver cells. Most enter erythrocytes from which up to 32 daughter cells are released after further parasitic cell division. The cycle continues, taking 2–3 days for the reproductive phase prior to reinfection of more erythrocytes. The characteristic bouts of fever occur at the same intervals as the parasites are liberated into the bloodstream. Eventually, sexual forms (gametocytes) arise which may be ingested by another mosquito whilst it feeds on blood from an infected person; the parasite's life-cycle then continues in the mosquito.

In tropical regions where malaria is endemic, the human population is exposed to the parasite from birth and considerable immunity develops, especially in black races. Interestingly, a gene whose possession leads to sickle cell anaemia also confers resistance to the most dangerous *Plasmodium* species.

Antimalarial drugs can be classifed by chemical structure (cinchona alkaloids, 4-aminoquinolines, 8-aminoquinolines), but it is helpful to use a classification based on the stage of the *Plasmodium* life-cycle which is most affected. First are the tissue schizonticides, like **primaquine**, which destroy the liver parasites soon after infection. Second are the blood schizonticides (**quinine, chloroquine, amodiaquine**), acting on the erythrocytic stage. Third are the sporonticides, like **proguanil** and **pyrimethamine**, which act slowly on several forms of the parasite and also inhibit later development in the mosquito. Fourth, a gametocidal action is seen with **primaquine**.

It should be emphasized that drug treatment is of great benefit to the individual with malaria, but that control of the vector (mosquito) may be a more effective method of combating the problem of malaria in a population as a whole.

In addition to its antimalarial uses, **chloroquine** is also employed as a second-line drug in patients with painful polyarthritis inadequately controlled by first-line non-steroidal anti-inflammatory agents. TTFFT

MCQ 188

Diseases caused by parasitic protozoan flagellates

1. include kala-azar, a visceral form of leishmaniasis.
2. often respond to aromatic diamidines like **pentamidine**.
3. include Chaga's disease, for which the drug of choice is **nifurtimox**.
4. may be treated with **mercaptopurine**.
5. include sleeping sickness, which is transmitted by tsetse flies.

Several tropical diseases are caused by protozoan flagellates of the genera *Trypanosoma* and *Leishmania*. Some complete their life-cycle in one host; others require two. Transmission to the human host is by insects, for example *Leishmania* by sand flies, *T. gambiense* and *T. rhodesiense* (causing sleeping sickness) by tsetse flies, and *T. cruzi* (causing Chaga's disease) by South American assassin bugs.

A greater occurrence of leishmaniasis has been noted in people living in temperate zones because many travel more widely for business or pleasure, but it is of great social and financial importance in areas where the parasite is endemic. Leishmaniasis exists in three clinical forms: a relatively mild, cutaneous one, a more disfiguring mucocutaneous infection (espundia) and a serious visceral disease (kala-azar), which is generally fatal if left untreated. In kala-azar, severe anaemia, muscle wasting, liver and spleen enlargement and prolonged fever occur. Immunological dysfunctions may permit opportunistic infections to take hold. Drug-resistant strains of *Leishmania* emerge in particular locations so treatment may vary between areas. Pentavalent antimonials (e.g. **sodium stibogluconate**) are the major drugs, while **amphotericin B** or **pentamidine** are more toxic substances which can be used in conjunction with antimonials or alone against antimony-resistant strains. Some drugs are being tested for topical application in the milder forms of leishmaniasis but their efficacy has not yet been proven.

Sleeping sickness occurs when some species of *Trypanosoma* penetrate the CNS. Patients are lethargic and apathetic, sleeping for long periods and becoming emaciated. Drugs of choice are the aromatic diamidines, which are taken up by the parasite and concentrated more than 1000-fold. **Pentamidine** is employed prophylactically as well as to treat an established infection but will only destroy those parasites in the bloodstream because it does not penetrate the CNS. Where parasites are lodged in the CNS or are resistant to **pentamidine**, arsenicals can be given but are toxic and only used in hospitals. The most common arsenical is a condensation product of the trivalent arsenical compound **melarsen oxide** with **dimercaprol**. The latter reduces the toxicity of **melarsen** to the patient but not to the trypanosome. **Dimercaprol** should not be confused with **mercaptopurine**, an anticancer drug acting at the stage of purine synthesis, used to treat leukaemias.

Chaga's disease (*T. cruzi*) affects cardiac and intestinal muscle. The drug of choice is **nifurtimox** but its usefulness is often outweighed by the severe neurological damage and allergic reactions which occur. TTTFT

Metronidazole

1. is an antifungal drug.
2. can eradicate *Trichomonas vaginalis* from females but not from males.
3. has been used in aversion therapy against **alcohol**.
4. is effective against several protozoal gut parasites like *Entamoeba*, *Giardia* and *Balantidia*.
5. may be used to treat Vincent's gingivitis.

Most diseases caused by protozoa are endemic in the tropics but some, for example amoebiasis, are common in temperate zones. A parasite like *Entamoeba* can be harboured without producing symptoms but carriers may pass the infection to others. Infection occurs when food or drink is contaminated with faecal material containing encysted *Entamoeba*. When the amoeba multiply in the gut, symptoms are produced which range from digestive upsets to severe intestinal ulceration, which may be fatal. Since the parasites can invade the intestinal wall or, via the bloodstream, reach the brain, lungs or liver, multiple drug therapy may be necessary.

Metronidazole is the drug of choice against amoebiasis. It is also effective against the protozoan parasites *Giardia* and *Balantidia* (intestinal) and *Trichomonas* (sexually transmitted, causing vaginitis in women and urethritis in men). **Metronidazole** has antibacterial activity, particularly against anaerobes. It is used to treat Vincent's disease caused by anaerobes infecting the gums. Within responsive microorganisms its nitro group is reduced and the reaction products kill the cells by interacting with a variety of macromolecules – an example of 'lethal synthesis'. In amoebiasis, **metronidazole** kills protozoa both in the lumen and in the gut wall but not encysted parasites. It is commonly prescribed with **diloxanide**, which affects only the luminal organisms. Tetracyclines are sometimes used in combination, especially in amoebic dysentery. Amoebic abscesses of the brain and liver may require the highly toxic **dehydroemetine** if they are to be eradicated, but this drug should only be used in hospital.

Against trichomoniasis, **metronidazole** is again the drug of choice. Females are most susceptible to infection after the menopause or after parturition since vaginal secretions are then nearer neutral pH (the normally acid conditions inhibit parasitization). **Metronidazole** should be given to both sexual partners even if the female alone requests treatment; often the disease is symptomless in the male. Candidiasis may occur in treated patients, who will then require antifungal therapy with drugs like **nystatin** or topical **amphotericin B**. Other unwanted effects of **metronidazole** include dizziness, ataxia, gastric upsets and skin rashes. **Metronidazole** also inhibits aldehyde dehydrogenase and allows ethanal to accumulate in the blood after drinking **ethanol**. This causes headache, vomiting and muscle pains and the drug has been used for aversion therapy in alcoholics to deter them from further drinking. FFTTT

MCQ 190

Antiviral effects may be produced by

1. immunological neutralization of the virus identified by its protein coat.
2. **amantadine** through the prevention of viral uncoating.
3. **acyclovir** through inhibition of DNA polymerase.
4. inhibition of reverse transcriptase in herpes viruses.
5. **azathioprine** through inhibition of reverse transcriptase.

Viruses consist of a core of nucleic acid (either DNA, e.g. herpes virus, or RNA in retroviruses such as human immunodeficiency virus; HIV) surrounded by a protein coat and in some cases an additional glycolipid membrane or envelope. They gain access to the body via for example the gastric, buccal or urogenital mucosa or through accidental (wounds) or intentional (injections) breaches in the skin. The virus may then encounter antibodies to the proteins of the virus coat/envelope. These antibodies may have arisen from previous exposure to the virus, from exposure to vaccines (e.g. polio, hepatitis, measles) or they can be purposely administered as a γ-globulin preparation (e.g. rubella) as a prophylactic measure. The presence of antibodies can be used as a diagnostic test (e.g. HIV).

The virus identifies its target cells by protein/glycoprotein molecules (receptors) on the cell membrane (e.g. CD4 protein for HIV). Antiviral therapy at this stage could involve: (a) blocking all the cell surface receptors, preventing binding of the virus; or (b) providing excess receptors, carried on suitable structures, with which the virus can combine harmlessly.

In the absence of such therapy, the virus fuses with and then enters the cell to be liberated from its coat by fusion with lysosomes. The low pH of the lysosome is essential to the uncoating process and **amantadine** has antiviral effects because it raises lysosomal pH and prevents uncoating. **Amantadine** is effective against influenza A but not against influenza B. Once uncoated, the nucleic acid of the virus (viral DNA or DNA derived from viral RNA by reverse transcriptase in the case of retroviruses) directs the protein synthesis mechanisms of the cell to produce new protein and the virus itself is replicated. The coat/envelope proteins and nucleic acid are assembled to produce new virus, which is released from the host cell by 'budding' or by disruption of the cell. Because the normal protein synthetic mechanisms of the host cell are involved and drugs usually exploit biochemical *differences* between cells, it is very difficult to discover a *selective* antiviral agent. However, the reverse transcriptase step in retroviruses is not involved in normal human cells and this constitutes a difference which may be exploited, for example in the treatment of AIDS with **azidothymidine (AZT;** not to be confused with the purine analogue **azathioprine)**.

Other antiviral mechanisms involve: (a) alteration in base-pairing properties to cause misreading/pairing of the sequence (**adenine arabinoside**); (b) inhibition of DNA or RNA polymerase. This enzyme allows a new base to be joined covalently to the end of a new growing strand of nucleic acid. The guanine analogue **acyclovir** is phosphorylated in virus-infected cells to a triphosphate form which inhibits DNA polymerase of the herpes virus when it attempts to use this analogue in place of the normal guanine deoxyribonucleoside triphosphate. TTTFF

Cancer Chemotherapy

MCQ 191

Neoplasms

1. include cancers of the bone marrow as well as solid tumours occurring in the viscera.
2. are carcinomas where there is no evidence of secondary growths.
3. should be treated with X-irradiation only if chemotherapy has been unsuccessful.
4. are highly susceptible to 'phase-specific' drugs when most of their stem cells are in phase G_0 of the cell cycle.
5. like Burkitt's lymphoma or chorioepithelioma may be completely cured by chemotherapy.

Cancer is a general term given to new growths of cells (neoplasms) which are no longer controlled in the normal way by the host. Cells may become detached from the original site and be carried by the lymphatic or blood vessels to other sites where they form secondary growths (metastases). Neoplasms are named according to the tissue from which the stem cells arise (e.g. carcinoma from epithelial tissue; sarcoma from connective tissue; lymphoma from lymphatic tissue). Unless the growth can be checked, some cancers will be fatal within weeks or years depending on the site of the growth and the rate of cell division. The host may die if some vital structure is invaded or if blood vessels are blocked. The growth of some cancers makes such a large demand on scarce body resources that general debilitation occurs, characterized by rapid weight loss, and death ensues.

Cancers can sometimes be eradicated by surgery (especially if removed before metastatic spread occurs) or by X-irradiation or by a combination of these physical approaches. Chemotherapy may be used in conjunction but can, by itself, bring about a cure (e.g. chorioepithelioma and Burkitt's lymphoma) or at least a prolonged remission (e.g. leukaemias and bone marrow neoplasms).

Drugs used to attack neoplasms are of two types: those which exert their toxic effect during a particular phase of the cell cycle (phase- or cycle-specific) and those which are not phase-specific. Before they can divide, cells synthesize DNA (phase S); they then enter the 'postsynthetic' period (G_2) during which synthesis of RNA and proteins occurs. Mitosis follows: a G_2 cell with a double complement of DNA gives rise to two daughter cells; these are in a 'presynthetic' phase (G_1), although enzymes are being produced, essential for the manufacture of DNA precursors. The daughter cells may immediately go through a similar cell cycle or enter a resting stage (G_0). For some specialized cells (e.g. neurones) no further division is possible, but slow-growing tumour cells may remain in G_0 for long periods before entering the cell cycle again. During their active periods cells are more susceptible to drugs which interfere with growth and division.

All cancers grow by division of their stem cells. In some solid tumours a large number of stem cells have irreversibly differentiated, are incapable of further division and can produce no further damage. By contrast, most forms of blood cell cancer have a high proportion of proliferating stem cells and these tend to be the most susceptible to chemotherapy. TFFFT

In the drug treatment of cancer

1. combinations of drugs may be used but only if all are chosen from the 'phase-specific' group.
2. alkylating agents can be employed which cause cross-linking of adjacent DNA strands in the nucleus.
3. substances like **melphalan** predominantly alkylate guanine molecules in nucleic acids.
4. **cyclophosphamide** and **chlorambucil** are both bis(chloroethyl)amine alkylating agents.
5. **metoclopramide** primarily alkylates thymidine residues.

Patients with overt signs of widespread cancer may have 10^{12} cancerous cells in the body. A drug which eliminates 99.9% of these cells will still leave 10^9 cells, most of them having the potential to divide and increase the malignancy. In many bacterial infections such a high 'kill rate' would end the infection by permitting natural defence mechanisms to cope with the survivors, but such mechanisms rarely appear to operate in human cancer. Kill rates of 100% are necessary and this may require long-term chemotherapy with combinations of drugs and procedures like X-irradiation.

It is common practice to combine drugs from each of the major groups (phase-specific and phase non-specific) to produce maximal effects. Therapy may involve up to four anticancer agents as well as other drugs (typically analgesics and also antiemetics like **chlorpromazine** and **metoclopramide**). The time at which phase-specific drugs are used is critical since they act only on stem cells which are passing through that particular phase of the cell cycle.

Many of the phase non-specific group are alkylating agents. Most have two (bis) active groups and this allows the cross-linking of alkylated cell components. These drugs evolved from the vesicant (blistering) sulphur-mustard and nitrogen-mustard gases produced during the two world wars. Examples are: bis(chloroethyl)amines like **cyclophosphamide**, **chlorambucil** and **melphalan**; the alkylsulphonate **busulphan**; and some nitrosoureas, such as **carmustine** (1, 3-bis(2-chloroethyl)-1-nitrosourea; BCNU), which are thought to act by carbamoylation as well as alkylation. All these agents can react with sulphydryl, hydroxyl and carboxyl groups, but are thought to be lethal to cancer cells by alkylating components of nuclear DNA. In the case of bis(chloroethyl)amine drugs, one chloroethylamine group cyclizes to the reactive etheniminium ion. This ion commonly alkylates bases of the DNA strands, reacting particularly with the nitrogen atom in guanine in position 7. Cross-linking of DNA strands will often occur when the second chloroethylamine group cyclizes and reacts with another base on an adjacent strand. The cytotoxicity results from the failure of cross-linked strands to separate prior to cell division, while sometimes base pairs become misaligned when one has been alkylated. These drugs are not phase-specific but cells are most susceptible in late G_1 and S phases, the cytotoxicity then being manifested in G_2, when the cell attempts to use the deformed DNA to synthesize RNA and protein. FTTTF

MCQ 193

Alkylating agents used in cancer chemotherapy

1. are limited mainly to the treatment of solid tumors.
2. often cause undesirable effects like vomiting, diarrhoea and headache.
3. include **busulphan**, given orally against chronic myelogenous leukaemia.
4. are no longer employed in Hodgkin's disease, which can now be cured surgically
5. include **cyclophosphamide**, which requires hepatic biotransformation to an active agent.

Alkylating agents generally produce headache, vomiting, diarrhoea and parasympathomimetic actions like salivation and bradycardia. Haemopoietic tissues are depressed and the leucocycte count may become very low. The particular sensitivity of the blood-forming tissue to these phase non-specific drugs explains their use against cancers caused by overactivity in these tissues.

The 'myeloproliferative' diseases are those in which bone marrow produces excessive blood cells, giving rise to various leukaemias or to polycythaemia. In the case of chronic myelogenous leukaemia (arising from a chromosomally abnormal haemopoietic cell) the most usual treatment is with **busulphan**, though other orally active alkylating agents may be used. Treatment may be intermittent, depending on the degree of depression of the white cell count, but resistance to the drug eventually develops. **Busulphan** causes little disturbance of the gastrointestinal tract and is well absorbed.

Reticuloses (e.g. Hodgkin's disease) arise from proliferation of reticulo-endothelial cells of the lymph nodes, spleen and bone marrow. Intensive X-irradiation is often curative especially in the early stages if the disease is confined to lymph nodes in just one region. In later stages an alkylating agent such as **mechlorethamine**, **chlorambucil** or **cyclophosphamide** is likely to be given as part of intensive combination therapy. **Cyclophosphamide** must be biotransformed by hepatic cytochrome P-450 mixed function oxidase systems to 4-hydroxycyclophosphamide and aldophosphamide, which are the active agents.

Nitrosoureas have also been used successfully against Hodgkin's disease and, in combination with other drugs, are often introduced when patients relapse or fail to respond to more common combinations. FTTFT

Of the various mechanisms by which anticancer drugs can affect pyrimidines

1. fluorodeoxyuridine prevents the formation of thymine.
2. **5-fluorouracil** is cytotoxic only after biotransformation to its mono-phosphate nucelotide.
3. **cytosine arabinoside** inhibits thymidylate synthetase.
4. both **5-fluorouracil** and **cytosine arabinoside** prevent cell division but permit synthesis of RNA and proteins to continue.
5. **azacytidine** is given orally and inhibits absorption of pyrimidines from the gut.

Just as inhibitors of purine synthesis have anticancer activity, so do drugs which block the formation of pyrimidine bases or their incorporation into DNA. **5-Fluorouracil** is one such drug and must be converted via its nucleo*side*, fluorodeoxyuridine (which has also been used as an anticancer drug), to its cytotoxic nucleo*tide*, fluorodeoxyuridine monophosphate. This derivative binds covalently to the thymidylate synthetase which catalyses the essential conversion of thymine to thymidine. The subsequent inhibition of DNA formation results in a 'thymine-less death' of cells since essentially the same effect would occur in cells deprived of thymine. **Methotrexate** also causes some blockade of thymidylate synthetase, although it is used mainly for its ability to block dihydrofolate reductase (and interferes with purine and pyrimidine synthesis by this latter mechanism).

Cytosine arabinoside acts during the S phase of the cell cycle only, being converted to the triphosphate derivative. This derivative blocks both DNA polymerase and the reductase responsible for the conversion of the essential cyt*idine* diphosphate to its deoxy- form. An incorporation of cyt*osine* arabinoside triphosphate into both DNA and RNA has been observed. The drug is used principally against myelogenous leukaemia.

Both **5-fluorouracil** and **cytosine arabinoside** exert their major toxic actions on the bone marrow and cause gastrointestinal disturbances. In general, their depressant action is on DNA formation, thereby stopping cell division, and they tend to permit both RNA formation and protein synthesis to continue unchecked.

A third drug in this group is **azacytidine**, which is converted to the monophosphate by uridine–cytidine kinase. The monophosphate inhibits orotydilate decarboxylase to reduce pyrimidine synthesis. Other metabolites of **azacytidine** become incorporated into DNA and RNA and so inhibit synthesis of nucleic acids as well as of proteins. It is a 'second-line' drug for acute leukaemia and must be given i.v. Undesirable effects are nausea and vomiting but it has been reported to cause profound depression of the bone marrow for long periods. FTFTF

MCQ 195

Of the cancer chemotherapeutic agents acting on purine synthesis

1. **mercaptopurine** irreversibly inhibits the enzyme which converts hypoxanthine to inosinic acid.
2. **6-thioguanine** is converted to 'false' thiol nucleotides which can become incorporated into DNA.
3. **mercaptopurine** becomes more toxic in the presence of **allopurinol**.
4. **azathioprine** must be biotransformed to **6-thioguanine** before it is active.
5. their principal toxic effects involve reductions in the number of circulating granulocytes and platelets.

Some phase-specific anticancer drugs act at the stage of purine synthesis. The first step in this reaction is the conversion of hypoxanthine to its ribonucleotide, inosinic acid, by hypoxanthine–guanine phosphoribosyl transferase (HGPT). **Mercaptopurine** resembles hypoxanthine chemically but has a sulphydryl (-SH) group instead of a hydroxyl. It is converted to 6-thioinosinic acid by HGPT, the 'false' product inhibiting several enzymes in the purine pathway *en route* to adenine and guanine nucleotides. In a similar manner, the corresponding sulphydryl analogue of guanine (**6-thioguanine**) also inhibits several enzymes in the pathway but requires deamination to form an active product. Thus purine thiols decrease guanine nucleotide levels generally and lead to the production of 'false' DNA and RNA which contain thiol groups.

Both **mercaptopurine** and **6-thioguanine** are absorbed from the gut and tend to be used against acute lymphatic leukaemia in adults and myeloid leukaemias in children. **Mercaptopurine** is biotransformed to an inactive product by xanthine oxidase and this enzyme is inhibited by **allopurinol**, which is often used as supportive therapy in some blood cancers. Soluble purines liberated from dying cancer cells are normally converted by xanthine oxidase to uric acid, an excess of which may cause gout or kidney damage. **Allopurinol** prevents the conversion, allowing the purines to be excreted unchanged. However, it also inhibits the biotransformation of **mercaptopurine**, the dose of which must be reduced.

Azathioprine, from which **mercaptopurine** is slowly released in the body, offers no advantage over **mercaptopurine** itself in the treatment of leukaemias. It is successfully used (often in combination with other immunosuppressive agents) in preventing rejection of transplanted tissue by suppression of lymphocyte proliferation. Its biotransformation, like that of **mercaptopurine**, is reduced by **allopurinol**.

The toxic effects of purine thiols are principally on the bone marrow, reducing the numbers of granulocytes and platelets in the blood. Less serious, but sometimes incapacitating, are the effects on the gastrointestinal tract like nausea, vomiting and diarrhoea. FTTFT

Some anticancer drugs are classified as 'antimetabolites'

1. because they inhibit the biotransformation of drugs whose metabolic products are carcinogenic.
2. and their inhibitory action results from alkylation of enzymes.
3. all of which are phase-specific.
4. like **methotrexate**, whose major action is to inhibit dihydrofolate reductase.
5. and are used only against cancer of the blood-forming tissues (e.g. against leukaemias).

The 'antimetabolites' form a large proportion of the phase-specific drugs. As their name implies, these drugs have chemical structures similar to precursors involved in the synthesis of nucleic acids and can, therefore, compete with them for the biosynthetic enzymes. Their mechanisms of action can vary; an antimetabolite may itself become converted to a 'false' precursor (e.g. **mercaptopurine**) or may cause irreversible blockade of an enzyme (e.g. **methotrexate**).

The most important biosynthetic reactions in cancer cells are those producing DNA, without the duplication of which the cells cannot divide. The synthesis of DNA begins with the production of purines (adenine and guanine) and pyrimidines (cytosine and thymine). Each of these bases is then linked to a pentose sugar forming a nucleo*side* to which is attached a molecule of phosphoric acid (to form a nucleo*tide*). When deoxy-ribonucleotides are joined to form a cross-linked chain, the resulting molecule is DNA, the major component of chromosomes. The unique order of the bases on the DNA strand represents the code which enables cells to duplicate themselves and also contains instructions for the cellular biosynthetic reactions. During phase G_1 of the cell cycle, enzymes are being produced which are essential for the production of DNA precursors and during phase S the DNA itself is synthesized. In both G and S phases, susceptibility to antimetabolites is high.

Folic acid is essential in dividing cells because it is converted via dihydrofolate (by dihydrofolate reductase) to tetrahydrofolic acid, which functions as a carrier of one-carbon fragments for use in the synthesis of purines and pyrimidines as well as some amino acids. Without these bases DNA synthesis cannot proceed. Neither can the synthesis of RNA and some proteins, all of which are dependent on tetrahydrofolate. **Methotrexate (amethopterin)** binds very tightly to the catalytic site on dihydrofolate reductase and thus blocks the enzymes. It can produce complete cure in cases of choriocarcinoma, though it may need to be given for more than a year and resistance to its effects may occur. **Methotrexate** has been used against many types of neoplasm, particularly leukaemias and carcinomas, either alone or in combination with other anticancer drugs. Its principal danger is bone marrow depression. FFTTF

MCQ 197

Naturally occurring products used as anticancer agents are

1. all phase-specific, disrupting cell division especially during phase G_0.
2. drugs like **vinblastine** and **vincristine**, which act by depolymerizing microtubules and so affect chromosomal distribution during mitosis.
3. drugs like **dactinomycin**, which intercalates between guanine and cytosine base pairs on DNA strands and inhibits subsequent RNA synthesis.
4. bleomycins, which bind to DNA and cause fragmentation of the strands.
5. substances such as **mitomycin**, one of the most active drugs against solid tumour stem cells which have adapted to a hypoxic environment.

Several naturally occurring products of plant or fungal origin are used to treat cancers. The alkaloids **vincristine** and **vinblastine** (from the periwinkle plant) have an unusual phase-specific action, working during mitosis. They are 'spindle poisons', binding to the microtubular protein tubulin, so that when the drug–tubulin complex is incorporated in the growing microtubule, depolymerization of the structure occurs. The segregation of chromosomes cannot take place in an orderly fashion and mitosis is arrested. **Vinblastine** is used to treat Hodgkin's disease and other lymphomas. **Vincristine** is used in acute leukaemia in children and in other rapidly dividing neoplasms. Its principal undesirable effect is peripheral neuritis though, like **vinblastine**, it sometimes produces bone marrow depression.

Bleomycins, from *Streptomyces verticillus*, are phase-specific. They bind to DNA, causing fragmentation of the chain and chromosomal abnormalities. Affected cells do not progress beyond the G_2 phase. Testicular and epithelial cancers are especially susceptible to **bleomycin** and it is sometimes used together with **vincristine** and **vinblastine**. A high incidence of fever has been reported as well as some lethal anaphylactic reactions. Pulmonary function is depressed but **bleomycin** causes little depression of the bone marrow.

Most of the other fungal products with anticancer activity are not phase-specific and they all appear to bind to a variety of components of DNA, thereby inhibiting DNA-directed RNA synthesis. **Daunorubicin** (antileukaemic) and the closely related **doxorubicin**, which acts against many types of neoplasm, are biotransformed by hepatic microsomal enzymes to active metabolites which intercalate between base pairs of DNA. **Dactinomycin** also intercalates between guanine and cytosine base pairs on adjacent strands of DNA. It is often used with **methotrexate** to treat choriocarcinoma. **Mithramycin** not only binds to DNA but also causes an unexpected calcium-lowering effect by an action of osteocytes and is used principally to reverse neoplastic hypercalcaemia. **Mitomycin** is converted into a polyfunctional alkylating agent by hepatic cytochrome P-450 reductase. It is one of the most active drugs against stem cells of solid tumours which have adapted to a hypoxic environment and, although rather toxic, is used increasingly in combination therapy. FTTTT

Particular neoplastic cells may be selectively inhibited by drugs: for example

1. cancers of thyroid follicular cells can be destroyed by **iodine-131** because they selectively accumulate **iodide.**
2. breast cancer cells with high levels of oestrogen receptors may be inhibited by large doses of oestrogen.
3. breast cancer cells with high levels of oestrogen receptors may be inhibited by antioestrogens like **tamoxifen.**
4. leukaemic cells with glucocorticoid receptors may be suppressed by **prednisolone.**
5. leukaemic cells with a poor capacity for synthesizing asparagine may regress if patients are given **asparaginase.**

Some types of neoplasm respond to treatment with steroids. Haematological cancers (leukaemias, lymphomas) are often treated with glucocorticoids like **prednisolone** or **dexamethasone** which suppress lymphocytic development and cause lymph node regression. These corticosteroids are nearly always used in combination therapy with phase-specific and phase non-specific drugs. Alternatively some solid tumours, for example prostatic cancers, respond to treatment with sex hormones; and some breast cancers often regress in the presence of large doses of oestrogens. Those cells which respond almost invariably have high levels of specific receptors for steroids. Biopsies may be performed in attempts to determine the receptor content of the neoplasm. Then it may be possible to predict which patients are most likely to respond favourably to treatment. It is known that the steroid hormone enters the target cell, binding to a soluble cytoplasmic receptor, which then undergoes transformation reactions (i.e. it fragments to produce a complex of lower molecular weight) before the steroid is translocated to the nucleus. Here, binding to DNA occurs to activate gene transcription.

It is not known why, in some patients, large doses of steroids cause tumour regression when the cells themselves are probably dependent on endogenous steroids (in lower concentrations) for their proliferation. However, of interest is the increasingly successful use of the *anti*oestrogen **tamoxifen** to treat breast tumours which contain cells with high levels of oestrogen receptors. Although more complex explanations have been advanced, the effectiveness has been attributed to a prevention of oestrogen access to the nuclei of cells that are dependent on the hormone for mitosis. Some prostatic cancers and endometrial cancers have responded favourably. **Tamoxifen,** given by mouth, lacks the toxic effects associated with either steroid therapy (mimicry and suppression of endogenous hormones) or most other anticancer drugs (bone marrow depression, gastrointestinal disturbances).

Other miscellaneous anticancer therapies include **asparaginase** and radioactive **iodine-131. Asparaginase** may be effective against acute leukaemia in childhood. The leukaemic cells require external **asparagine**, whilst normal cells will synthesize their own. The enzyme reduces plasma levels so that less amino acid is taken up and protein synthesis is thereby inhibited. Thyroid follicular cell carcinoma may be treated with **iodine-131** as **sodium iodide** ($Na^{131}I$), a β- and γ-emitter with a half-life of 8 days. The material is avidly taken up by the cells and, therefore, produces a selective destruction by β-irradiation. TTTTT

Index of Drug Names

Note: the numbers referred to in the index are those of the relevant MCQs.

α-Methyldopa 61, 82, 86
αβ-Methylene ATP 71
Methylthiouracil 174
α-Methyl-p-tyrosine 61
Methysergide 72, 121
Metiamide 112
Metoclopramide 113, 150, 192
Metoprolol 84
Metronidazole 101, 189
Metyrapone 170
Mianserin 156, 157, 160
Midazolam 138, 139
Minoxidil 82
Mithramycin 197
Mitomycin 197
Morphine 5, 15, 27, 121, 150, 162, 163, 164, 166
Muscarine 41, 43
Muscimol 128, 138

Naloxone 164
Naltrexone 164
Naphazoline 64
Neomycin 28, 182
Neostigmine 42, 48, 49, 50, 132
Nerve growth factor antiserum 63
Nialamide 159, 160
Nicotine 41, 58, 165
Nifedipine 80, 82, 85, 88, 91, 95
Nifurtimox 188
Nitrazepam 130, 138, 139, 143, 145
Nitroglycerin (glyceryl trinitrate) 1, 78, 89, 94
Nitroprusside 78, 82, 94
Nitrous oxide 134, 135
Noradrenaline 29, 35, 36, 43, 58, 63, 64, 65, 75
Norethisterone 169
Norgesterol 169
Normetanephrine 62
Nortriptyline 156
Nystatin 189

17-β-Oestradiol 62, 68
Ouabain 4, 96, 97
Oxacillin 179, 186
Oxazepam 145
Oxymetazoline 64
Oxytetracycline 181, 182

Pancuronium 28, 46, 48, 132
Papaverine 162
Paracetamol 164
Paraoxon 13
Parathion 13
Pargyline 62, 159, 160

Pempidine 44, 45, 86
Penicillamine 155
Penicillin 8, 26, 28, 178, 179, 180
Pentagastrin 112
Pentamethonium 57
Pentamidine 188
Pentazocine 16, 164
Pentobarbitone 136
Perchlorate 174
Pertussis toxin 68
Pethidine 27, 164
Phenelzine 27, 160
Phenformin 177
Phenobarbitone 17, 29, 136, 142, 143, 145
Phenolphthalein 166
Phenoxybenzamine 64, 72, 95
Phentolamine 64, 72
Phenylephrine 64, 65, 69, 70, 75
Phenytoin (diphenylhydantoin) 91, 112, 141, 142
Pholcodine 164, 166
Phthalylsulphathiazole 183
Physostigmine 49, 50, 51, 54, 57, 158
Picrotoxin 128
Pilocarpine 41, 43, 54
Pimozide 151
Pirenzepine 41, 52, 53, 56, 112, 113
Piretanide 83
Platelet activating factor (PAF) 109
Potassium chloride 28, 35
Practolol 74
Pralidoxime 49
Prazosin 64, 71, 72, 75, 82, 85, 95
Prednisolone 27, 123, 125, 172, 198
Prenylamine 80
Prilocaine 38, 39
Primaquine 187
Proadifen (SKF-525A) 17
Procainamide 91, 92
Procaine 73
Prochlorperazine 150
Proguanil 187
Promazine 29, 150
Promethazine 111, 148, 150
Propranolol 7, 12, 14, 33, 73, 74, 75, 84, 85, 88, 91, 92, 174
Propylthiouracil 17
Prostacyclin (prostaglandin I_2) 103
Protamine 102, 176
Puromycin 117
Pyridostigmine 50
Pyrimethamine 187

Quinidine 91, 92, 93
Quinine 187
Quisqualate 128